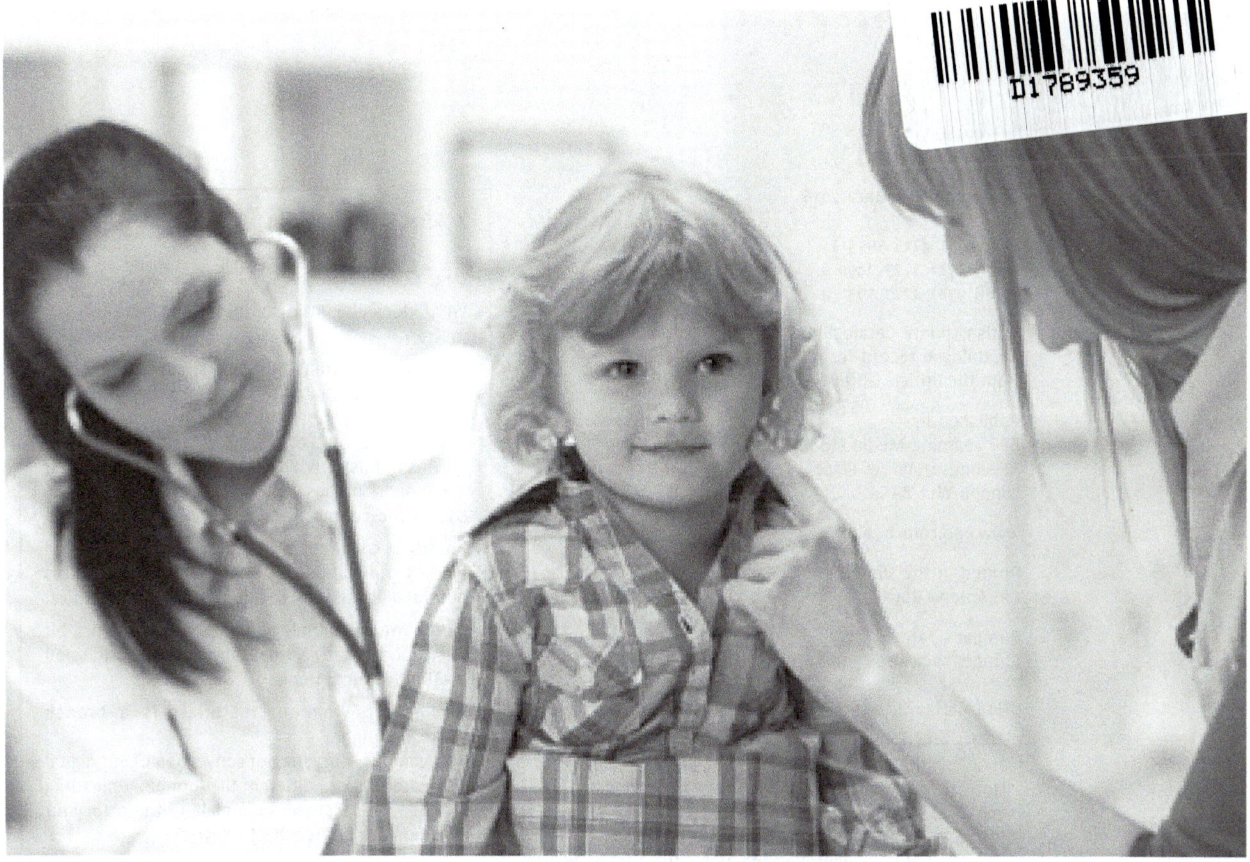

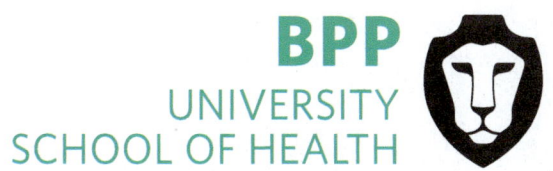

BMJ Easily Missed?:

Children and young people

Edited by
Professor Anthony Harnden & Dr Richard Lehman

BPP
UNIVERSITY
SCHOOL OF HEALTH

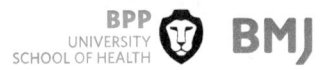

First edition January 2016

ISBN 9781 4727 3913 1
eISBN 9781 4727 4499 9
eISBN 9781 4727 3938 4

British Library Cataloguing-in-Publication Data
A catalogue record for this book is available
from the British Library

Published by
BPP Learning Media Ltd
BPP House, Aldine Place
London W12 8AA

www.bpp.com/health

Printed in the United Kingdom by
CPI Antony Rowe

Bumper's Farm,
Chippenham,
Wiltshire
SN14 6LH

Your learning materials, published by BPP Learning Media
Ltd, are printed on paper sourced from sustainable,
managed forests.

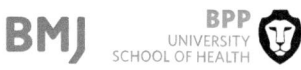

About the publisher

BPP Learning Media is dedicated to supporting aspiring professionals with top quality learning material. BPP Learning Media's commitment to success is shown by our record of quality, innovation and market leadership in paper-based and e-learning materials. BPP Learning Media's study materials are written by professionally-qualified specialists who know from personal experience the importance of top quality materials for success.

About The BMJ

The BMJ (formerly the British Medical Journal) in print has a long history and has been published without interruption since 1840. The BMJ's vision is to be the world's most influential and widely read medical journal. Our mission is to lead the debate on health and to engage, inform, and stimulate doctors, researchers, and other health professionals in ways that will improve outcomes for patients. We aim to help doctors to make better decisions. BMJ, the company, advances healthcare worldwide by sharing knowledge and expertise to improve experiences, outcomes and value.

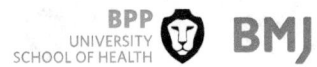

Contents

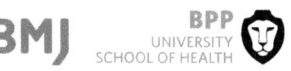

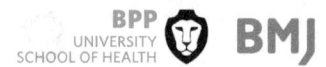

About the editors

Professor Anthony Harnden is an academic general practitioner at the University of Oxford who has worked five clinical sessions as a partner in general practice in Wheatley, Oxfordshire for more than 25 years. He has published original research papers in general practice related topics, with a focus on children. Professor Harnden is a Deputy Chairman of the Joint Committee of Vaccination and Immunisation (JCVI) and has been responsible for advising the UK government on vaccine policy since 2006. He was the primary care lead for the UK Confidential Enquiry into Child Deaths (2004-8), chaired a group to write a national Royal College of General Practitioners Child Health Strategy (2010-15) and developed the successful series 'Easily Missed?' in The BMJ (2009-).

Dr Richard Lehman is Senior Advisory Fellow in General Practice at the UK Cochrane Centre. He was a full-time general practitioner in Banbury for 32 years. For the last 17 years he has also written a weekly summary of the principal medical journals which is posted on The BMJ website. After retirement from UK general practice in 2010 he has worked on studies of the patient experience, and has spent a year at Yale working with the Yale University Open Data Access (YODA) project and remains a consultant to the group. His main interest is in ways to develop better informed dialogue with patients and he is on the steering committees of the NICE shared decision making initiative and Academy of Medical Royal Colleges Choosing Wisely group.

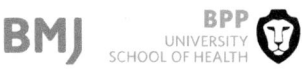

Foreword

I remember reading Sir Roy Meadow's 'Lecture Notes on Paediatrics' as a medical student. This contained an appendix attributed to Professor Ronald Illingworth which set out how many years the average general practitioner would have to be in practice to encounter some of the conditions described in the book. For example, a disease such as cystic fibrosis, which to a paediatrician seems common and which all medical students will be taught about, affects approximately 1 in 2,500 children born in the UK. An average GP with an average patient list of 2000 people today would expect there to be 10-15 pregnancies per annum arising from this cohort. On average, therefore, a new case of cystic fibrosis would occur once in the GP's list once every 150-250 years. For Hirschsprung's disease, one of the conditions covered in 'Easily Missed', Professor Illingworth estimated a British GP would have to be in practice for 600 years to see a child presenting with this condition!

In the UK, a GP list of 2000 patients would include about 400 patients under the age of 18 and these children and young people might account for 25% of consultations. Nevertheless, the concept of "easily missed" is not difficult to appreciate. I agree with Sir William Osler who said that "To study the phenomena of disease without books is to sail an uncharted sea, while to study books without patients is not to go to sea at all". However, it must be obvious from the frequency of rare conditions and an average of eight weeks of child health in the undergraduate curriculum that the future GP is reliant on books with so much uncharted sea. This is where 'Easily Missed' sits.

The GP also faces two other impediments which the hospital paediatrician does not. Firstly, the GP is the initial point of contact for families and research has shown that GP's deal with 90% of children's complaints, both in office hours and at nights and weekends. Inevitably, therefore, they see many minor problems and the challenge is to spot the serious needle in the haystack of often mild and self-limiting illness. In contrast, the consultant paediatrician has the benefit of primary care as their 'gatekeeper' or filter and there is therefore a greater likelihood that any child referred for a hospital outpatient appointment does have a more significant problem. Secondly, with inpatients the paediatrician has the luxury of daily review and a team of children's nurses and trainee paediatricians to discuss the case with. The GP is seeing the child at a snapshot in time during a very short consultation. Whilst the case can be discussed with partners and reviewed at another appointment, this is not the same as a hospital paediatric team consulting together in real time.

With the exception of cow's milk allergy and joint hypermobility, all of the conditions in this book are rather rare and therefore certainly "easily missed". The consequences of missing some of these conditions, even briefly, could be life threatening – for example coarctation of the aorta in a newborn or imported malaria. In others, the consequences are less acute but no less serious. For example, all the evidence is that the Kasai operation for biliary atresia is much more likely to have a good outcome if the diagnosis is made promptly and surgery completed by eight weeks of age. I am sure this book will help the reader avoid missing any of the conditions which 'Easily Missed' covers.

Professor Terence Stephenson

BSc, DM, FRCPCH, FRCP, FRACP, FRCPI, FRCS, FHKAP, FRCGP, FRCA, FCAI

Nuffield Professor of Child Health, Institute of Child Health, UCL and Honorary Consultant Paediatrician, University College Hospital and Great Ormond Street Hospital, London

Past President, Royal College of Paediatrics and Child Health

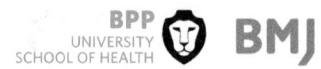

Introduction to Easily Missed series

Patients consult doctors with the expectation of an accurate diagnosis and advice on treatment. But in primary care, patients often present with undifferentiated symptoms without an immediately apparent diagnosis. For most conditions this doesn't matter because the symptoms either resolve or become worse in such a way that the patient returns before any harm is done. In consultations, general practitioners work by using the probability that the collection of presenting symptoms reflects a specific diagnosis. A combination of knowledge, clinical experience, and sound judgment ensures that they usually get it right.

The BMJ series "Easily Missed?" has raised awareness among general practitioners of conditions that are under-recognised in primary care at first presentation. The series has included a wide range of conditions, including some that are common but under-diagnosed and others that are uncommon but so serious that they need to be thought of whenever there is any possibility of their existence.

The articles are short and focused on diagnosis at presentation rather than treatment. The conditions described fulfil four key criteria. Firstly, there is evidence that the condition is commoner than most general practitioners realise or is often missed at first presentation. Secondly, the condition is sufficiently common that the average full time general practitioner in the UK will encounter it at least once a year, or else be so serious that delayed diagnosis is likely to worsen prognosis substantially. Thirdly, the condition has easily defined diagnostic features or diagnostic tests with known predictive characteristics. Fourthly, and most importantly, timely recognition will benefit the patient.

Judging from online access, the series has proved popular amongst readers of The BMJ. We hope that many patients have received early and insightful diagnoses as a result. The series would not have been possible without the dedication, hard work and wisdom of our in house editor, Dr Mabel Chew. She has been a delight to work with and we are very grateful for all her efforts.

Osler said "Medicine is a science of uncertainty and an art of probability." Although uncertainty will always be with us in primary care, the series might teach us more about the art of probability.

Anthony Harnden and Richard Lehman

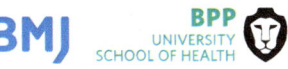

Coarctation of the aorta in the newborn

Mallika Punukollu, general practitioner[1],
Anthony Harnden, university lecturer in general practice[2],
Robert Tulloh, consultant, reader in paediatric cardiology[3]

[1]Kershaw Unit, Gartnavel Royal Hospital, Glasgow G12 0XH, UK

[2]Department of Primary Health Care, University of Oxford, Oxford OX3 7LF, UK

[3]Bristol Congenital Heart Centre, University Hospitals Bristol NHS Foundation Trust, Bristol BS2 8BJ, UK

Correspondence to: M Punukollu mpunukollu@gmail.com

Cite this as: BMJ 2011;343:d6838

DOI: 10.1136/bmj.d6838

www.bmj.com/content/343/bmj.d6838

Case scenario

A 14 day old infant presented with poor feeding, sleepiness, and loss of weight. He was born at term with normal vaginal delivery and was discharged within 24 hours after a newborn check was normal. Examination showed mild tachycardia, tachypnoea, weak femoral pulses, and a soft systolic murmur at the left sternal edge. The lungs were clear and the liver was enlarged by 3 cm. He was immediately referred to a specialist paediatric cardiology centre, where, after further investigation, a diagnosis of coarctation of the aorta was confirmed, prostaglandin was started, and the patient had successful surgical correction.

What is coarctation of the aorta?

Congenital heart disease is the commonest group of congenital diseases. It affects 19 in 1000 live births worldwide[1] and accounts for 9% of infant deaths in the United Kingdom.[2] Coarctation of the aorta is a discrete narrowing of the proximal descending aorta and accounts for 7% of congenital heart defects (figs 1 to 3).[1][3]

Why is coarctation of the aorta missed?

Coarctation of the aorta is the most commonly missed congenital heart disease,[3][4] and many cases not diagnosed until adulthood or death are incorrectly attributed to sepsis.[1]

Coarctation of the aorta may be missed in newborns because of the low sensitivity (32%) of the neonatal screening examination.[5] Moreover, cardiac symptoms may not develop before 48 hours of age and closure of the patent ductus arteriosus (fig 3).[3][6]

Other factors contributing to a delay in diagnosis include a lack of familiarity by clinicians with the clinical manifestations of coarctation of the aorta; 20% of babies with coarctation in the UK are undiagnosed at the 6-8 week examination.[7] One study found that only 56% of eligible babies had a routine examination for signs of heart disease between 6 and 8 weeks of age, and even if an abnormality was suspected there were delays in referral. In another study about a quarter of babies with murmurs had structural heart disease but only about half were referred.[8] In babies with coarctation of the aorta, 25-85% are estimated to have a bicuspid aortic valve.[9][10][11] In addition, they may have other associated cardiovascular abnormalities, such as ventricular septal defect (in 15% of cases) and persistent ductus arteriosus (13%).[11]

KEY POINTS

- Suspected congenital heart disease in the newborn is a medical emergency
- Coarctation of the aorta is the most commonly missed congenital heart disease
- Remain alert for the possibility of coarctation of the aorta, especially in an infant presenting with poor feeding, failure to thrive, or signs of heart failure
- Specific physical findings include a systolic murmur, weak or absent femoral pulses, and upper body hypertension
- However, a normal result on examination of a newborn does not rule out congenital heart disease
- Detection and treatment of coarctation of the aorta reduces morbidity and mortality from heart failure and improves long term outcome

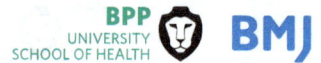

> **HOW COMMON IS COARCTATION OF THE AORTA?**
>
> - Coarctation of the aorta occurs in 1 per 2000-2500 live births worldwide[1]
> - It is the sixth most common form of congenital heart disease[1]

Why does this matter?

Suspected congenital heart disease is a medical emergency. Thirty infants a year in California, USA, die of a missed or late diagnosis of critical congenital heart disease.[3] A retrospective cohort study of 898 infants who died with congenital heart disease found that more than half of them died at home or in the emergency department and that coarctation of the aorta and hypoplastic left heart syndrome were the most commonly missed diagnoses and were associated with the highest mortality.[3] Coarctation of the aorta was missed in 27% of missed cases of congenital heart diseases (n=152) with mean age at death 17 days.[3] Studies have found that many of the complications (such as hypertension, coronary artery disease, congestive heart failure, recoarctation, aortic aneurysm, aortic rupture, and cerebrovascular accidents[9] [10] [11]) caused by delayed referral of children with coarctation of the aorta could have been prevented if the clinician had checked for the presence of femoral pulses,[4] which is recommended by guidelines from England's National Institute for Health and Clinical Excellence as part of the routine neonatal examination.[12]

Early diagnosis of coarctation of the aorta reduces morbidity and mortality from heart failure[13] and is critical for the proper timing of therapeutic interventions. The repair of coarctation of the aorta during early childhood is associated with less systemic hypertension and improved long term outcome.[9] [10] [11]

How is coarctation of the aorta diagnosed?

Clinical features

Infants may be asymptomatic until closure of the ductus arteriosus. After closure detectable physical signs (hypertension and/or abnormal femoral pulse) develop by 5 days of age, and almost half of the children affected will develop severe symptoms before 14 days of age

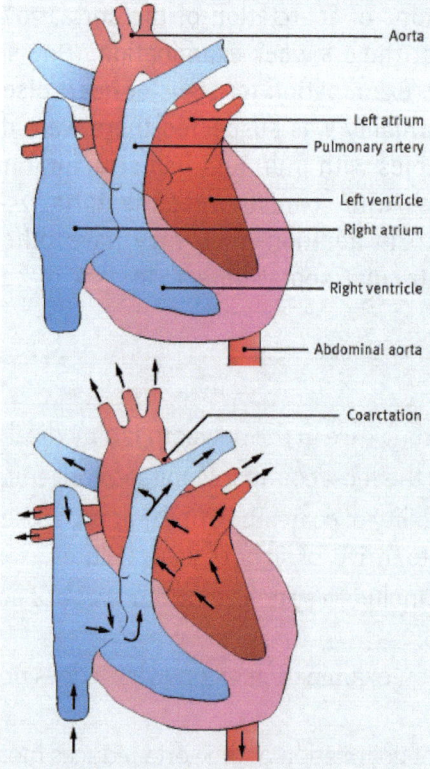

Fig 1 Top: Normal heart. Bottom: Heart with coarctation of the aorta (arrows indicate direction of all blood flow)

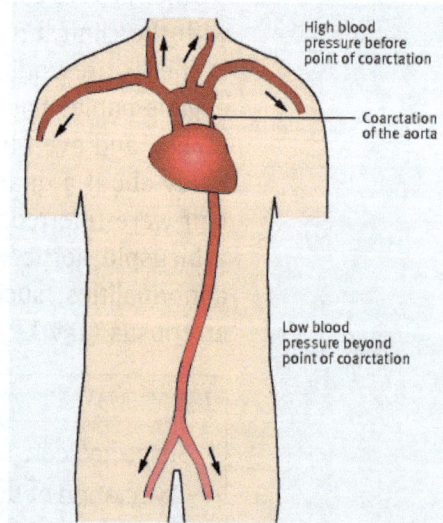

Fig 2 Coarctation of the aorta is a narrowing of the aorta, the major artery leading from the heart to the body. Blood pressure above the constriction is high, leading to upper limb hypertension. Below the constriction the blood pressure is low, causing poor perfusion and symptoms such as leg fatigue, cold feet, and weak femoral pulses

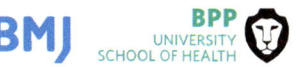

(that is, before the first vaccination visit).[6] Infants may develop poor feeding, tachypnoea, cool legs and feet, and pale or possibly grey skin discoloration. These signs may reflect heart failure and cardiogenic shock.[14] A retrospective study of 165 infants with congenital heart disease found that the commonest symptoms were breathlessness (75%), lower respiratory tract infections (45%), and failure to thrive (39%).[15] Coarctation of the aorta may cause faltering growth because of breathlessness (causing poor feeding and low energy intake) and in some cases high energy requirements (causing insufficient energy for normal growth).[16]

Older children and adults may have exercise intolerance; symptoms of poor perfusion such as leg fatigue, cold feet, and claudication; headache (resulting from hypertension); and symptoms of heart failure.[14]

A harsh systolic murmur (often absent in newborns) over the left sternal border indicates a 54% chance of an underlying cardiac malformation.[17] Weak or absent femoral pulses are found in 92% of infants with coarctation of the aorta,[18] and in these cases referral should be made to a paediatrician for blood pressure measurements. Upper limb hypertension has been found in 97% of infants with coarctation of the aorta[18] and a systolic blood pressure that is ≥20 mm Hg higher in the arms than in the legs is evidence of coarctation of the aorta (specificity 92%).[19] However, a negative finding on the four limb blood pressure measurement does not exclude the condition.[19]

Investigations

Pulse oximetry in the feet can detect 92% of duct dependent congenital heart disease (coarctation of the aorta, transposition of the great arteries, and hypoplastic left heart syndrome) and has a very low false positive rate (0.17%).[20] In addition, it is easy to use, reliable, and cost effective.[20]

Imaging and haemodynamic evaluation by transthoracic echocardiography is the recommended investigation to confirm the type of congenital heart disease.[21] Transthoracic echocardiography has a sensitivity of 91% in detecting coarctation of the aorta and 100% for all cardiac defects.[22]

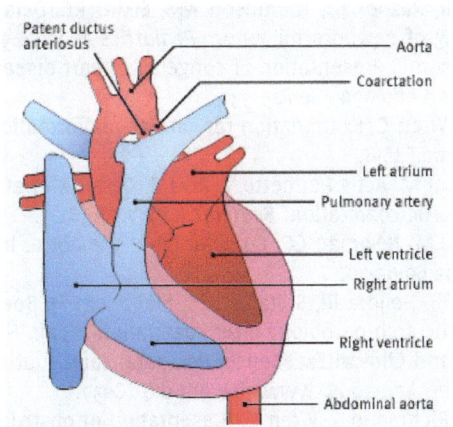

Fig 3 Heart with coarctation of the aorta and patent ductus arteriosus. Blood flow is restricted through the coarctation but can flow through the open connection between the aorta and the pulmonary artery, the ductus arteriosus. Symptoms usually do not occur until the ductus closes, usually when the newborn is a few days to about 2 weeks old. After the closure, the blood supplied through the ductus stops causing an increase in afterload on the heart leading to heart failure, and low blood pressure can result

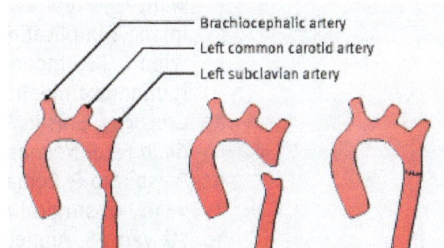

Fig 4 Surgical management of coarctation of the aorta: resection with end to end anastomosis

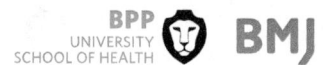

How is coarctation of the aorta managed?

The initial treatment, after resuscitation of the neonate, would involve the use of prostaglandin to reopen the arterial duct.[23] This usually leads to stabilisation, often in conjunction with intensive care support. Surgical repair usually takes place within a few days of presentation (fig 4).

In older children, control hypertension after surgery with β blockers, angiotensin converting enzyme inhibitors, or angiotensin receptor blockers as first line medications. In coarctation of the aorta, stent insertion at cardiac catheterisation has become the treatment of first choice in older children and in adults. This is most appropriate when there is a localised narrowing at the site of the coarctation, rather than a hypoplastic arch, which might require surgery.[24]

Long term follow-up postoperatively is mandatory because of the risk of systemic hypertension, aneurysm formation, or emergence of symptoms associated with congenital heart disease.

Contributors: MP wrote the first draft of the article, which was modified by AH and RT. All authors agreed the final draft.

Funding: None.

Competing interests: All authors have completed the ICMJE uniform disclosure form at www.icmje. org/coi_disclosure.pdf (available on request from the corresponding author) and declare: no support from any organisation for the submitted work; no financial relationships with any organisations that might have an interest in the submitted work in the previous three years; no other relationships or activities that could appear to have influenced the submitted work.

Provenance and peer review: Not commissioned; externally peer reviewed.

Patient consent not required (patient anonymised, dead, or hypothetical).

1   Hoffman JIE, Kaplan S. The incidence of congenital heart disease. *J Am Coll Cardiol* 2002;39:1890-900.
2   Abu-Harb M, Hey E, Wren C. Death in infancy from unrecognised congenital heart disease. *Arch Dis Child* 1994;71:3-7.
3   Rueny-Kang R. Chang, Gurvitz M, Rodriguez S. Missed diagnosis of critical congenital heart disease. *Arch Pediatr Adolesc Med* 2008;162:969-74.
4   Massin MM, Dessy H. Delayed recognition of congenital heart disease. *Postgrad Med J* 2006;82:468-70.
5   Knowles R, Griebsch I, Dezateux C, Brown J, Bull C, Wren C. Newborn screening for congenital heart defects: a systematic review and cost-effectiveness analysis. *Health Technol Assess* 2005;9:1-152, iii-iv.
6   Ward KE, Pryor RW, Matson JR, Razook JD, Thompson WM, Elkins RC. Delayed detection of coarctation in infancy: implication for timing of newborn follow-up. *Pediatrics* 1990;86:972-6.
7   Wren C, Richmond S, Donaldson L. Presentation of congenital heart disease in infancy: implications for routine examination. *Arch Dis Child* 1999;80:F49-53.
8   Gregory J, Emslie A, Wyllie J, Wren C. Examination for cardiac malformations at six weeks of age. *Arch Dis Child Fetal Neonatal Ed* 1999;80:F46-8.
9   Presbitero P, Demarie D, Villani M, Actis Perinetto V, Riva G, Orzan F, et al. Long term results (15 to 30 years) of surgical repair of aortic coarctation. *Br Heart J* 1987;57:462-7.
10 Stewart AB, Ahmed R, Travill CM, Newman CG. Coarctation of the aorta, life and health 20-44 years after surgical repair. *Br Heart J* 1993;69:65-70.
11 Roos-Hesselink JW, Schölzel BE, Heijdra RJ, Spitaels SEC, Meijboom FJ, Boersma E, et al. Congenital heart disease: aortic valve and aortic arch pathology after coarctation repair. *Heart* 2003;89:1074-7.
12 National Institute for Health and Clinical Excellence. Postnatal care: routine postnatal care of women and their babies. (Clinical guideline 37.) 2006. www.nice.org.uk/CG037.
13 Abu-Harb M, Wyllie J, Hey E, Richmond S, Wren C. Presentation of obstructive left heart malformations in infancy. *Arch Dis Child Fetal Neonatal Ed* 1994;71:F179-83.
14 Rao PS. Coarctation of the aorta. *Curr Cardiol Rep* 2005;7:425-34.
15 Tank S, Malik S, Joshi S. Epidemiology of congenital heart disease among hospitalised patients. *Bombay Hospital Journal* 2004;46(2):141-5.
16 Menon G, Poskit EME. Why does congenital heart disease cause failure to thrive? *Arch Dis Child* 1985;60:1134-9.
17 Ainsworth SB, Wyllie JP, Wren C. Murmurs in neonates. *Arch Dis Child Fetal Neonatal Ed* 1999;80:F43-5.
18 Ing FF, Starc TJ, Griffths SP, Gersony M. Early diagnosis of coarctation of the aorta in children: a continuing dilemma. *Pediatrics* 1996;98:378-82.
19 Crossland DS, Furness JC, Abu-Harb M, Sadagopan SN, Wren C. Variability of four limb blood pressure in normal neonates. *Arch Dis Child Fetal Neonatal Ed* 2004;89:F325-7.

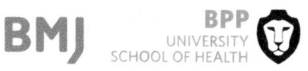

20 Granelli AD, Wennergren M, Sandberg K, Mellander M, Bejlum C, Inganäs L, et al. Impact of pulse oximetry screening on the detection of duct dependent congenital heart disease: a Swedish prospective screening study in 39821 newborns. *BMJ* 2009;338:a3037.

21 Warnes CA, Williams RG, Bashore TM, Child JS, Connolly HM, Dearani JA, et al. American College of Cardiology/American Heart Association 2008 guidelines for the management of adults with congenital heart disease: an executive summary. *Circulation* 2008;118:e714-833.

22 Türkvatan A, Akdur PO, Olçer T, Cumhur T. Coarctation of the aorta in adults: preoperative evaluation with multidetector CT angiography. *Diagn Interv Radiol* 2009;15:269-74.

23 Gersony WM, Peckham GJ, Ellison RC, Miettinen OS, Nadas AS. Effects of indomethacin in premature infants with patent ductus arteriosus: results of a national collaborative study. J Pediatr 1983;102:895-906.

24 Deanfield J, Thaulow E, Warnes C, Webb G, Kolbel F, Hoffman A, et al. Management of grown up congenital heart disease. *Eur Heart J* 2003;24:1035-84.

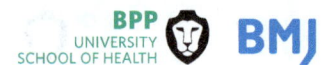

Biliary atresia

Jane Hartley, consultant paediatric hepatologist[1],
Anthony Harnden, university lecturer[2],
Deirdre Kelly, consultant paediatric hepatologist[1]

[1]Birmingham Children's Hospital, Birmingham B4 6NH

[2]Department of Primary Health Care, Oxford University, Oxford OX3 7LF

Correspondence to: J Hartley Jane.Hartley@bch.nhs.uk

Cite this as: BMJ 2010;340:c2383

DOI: 10.1136/bmj.c2383

www.bmj.com/content/340/bmj.c2383

Biliary atresia is a rare (one in 17000 in the United Kingdom[1]) but serious liver disorder that presents with jaundice in the first few weeks of life in apparently well infants. About 50 cases of biliary atresia occur each year in term babies who are born healthy and have usually had normal antenatal scans.[2] The lumen of the biliary tree is obliterated by an inflammatory cholangiopathy, which obstructs the flow of bile from the liver to the intestine, resulting in progressive liver damage. Early surgery to reconstruct the biliary tree may reduce further damage and prevent the need for liver transplantation.

Why is it missed?

The diagnosis of neonatal liver disease, including biliary atresia, may be missed because of confusion with either physiological jaundice or breast milk jaundice (which is common and is thought to occur in as many as 60% of normal term infants[3]). Physiological jaundice should last only for two to three days in term infants, whereas breast milk jaundice can last for as long as 12 weeks.[4] Both forms of jaundice are associated with a rise in unconjugated bilirubin.

Prolonged jaundice, which persists beyond 14 days in term infants and 21 days in preterm infants, requires further investigation for a pathological cause, even if the mother is breast feeding.

Most infants with biliary atresia will appear well in the first few weeks of life, and there is usually no family history of liver disease.

Why does this matter?

The restoration of bile flow from the liver to the bowel is essential to prevent further scarring of the liver. This requires a palliative Roux-en-Y portojejunostomy, known as a Kasai procedure. The earlier the Kasai procedure is carried out, the more likely it is to be successful (defined as a normal bilirubin concentration within 6 months of the procedure) with 60% of babies achieving good bile flow.[5] The diagnosis is made very late (beyond 100 days of age) in about 8% of cases[6]; when the diagnosis is this late, a Kasai procedure is unlikely to be successful owing to advanced liver damage or cirrhosis. In children who present late or in whom the operation is unsuccessful (the success rate decreases with increasing age at the time of the Kasai procedure[7]), liver transplantation within the first year of life is the only option.

> **KEY POINTS**
>
> - In any term infant with jaundice that persists beyond 2 weeks of age examine the colour of the stools and urine and refer for urgent measurement of the concentration of conjugated bilirubin (normal <20 μmol/l)
> - An early diagnosis of biliary atresia facilitates a successful Kasai portoenterostomy, with 60% of babies achieving good bile flow, which delays the need for liver transplantation
> - The late diagnosis of biliary atresia, an unsuccessful Kasai procedure, or advancing liver disease despite a successful Kasai (such as secondary to recurrent ascending cholangitis) requires lifesaving liver transplantation in infancy

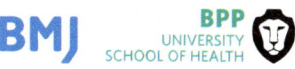

CASE SCENARIO

A mother presents to her general practitioner with her 3 week old son with mild jaundice; he is her first baby and fully breastfed. The mother was reassured. At the examination at age 8 weeks, the GP notices he has mildly icteric sclera and, on questioning, the mother states that his stools are cream coloured and his urine very yellow. The GP immediately refers the infant to the local paediatric unit, where further testing shows conjugated bilirubin concentrations of 120 μmol/l and leads to a final diagnosis of biliary atresia. The Kasai portoenterostomy carried out at age 9 weeks was unsuccessful, and he had a liver transplant at age 6 months.

HOW COMMON IS IT?

- Biliary atresia is the most common indication for liver transplantation in childhood

- The younger the baby at the time of a Kasai portoenterostomy, the more likely the procedure is to be successful and avoid the need for liver transplantation

- When the diagnosis of biliary atresia is made very late (beyond 100 days of age) children usually need a liver transplant in the first year of life

How is it diagnosed?

Clinical features

On examination the baby will have icteric sclera but will usually appear well unless the diagnosis is delayed, when signs of chronic liver disease (hepatomegaly, excessive bruising, ascites, and splenomegaly) will become obvious. Biliary atresia can occur in preterm infants, and in 20% of all cases biliary atresia is associated with cardiac malformations, polysplenia, and situs inversus, which will be identified on ultrasound scan.[8] The baby may be excessively hungry as a result of the poor absorption of long chain fat (secondary to the lack of bile in the intestine) and the high catabolic demand of liver disease.

Investigations

In all term babies with prolonged jaundice examine the colour of the stool and urine.[9] During the neonatal period the colour of stools varies but will become gradually paler in infants with biliary atresia,[10] and the urine colour will be yellow (it is normally colourless). Refer the infant to a local paediatric unit for a split bilirubin blood test (measuring conjugated and unconjugated bilirubin). Infants with prolonged physiological jaundice or prolonged breast milk jaundice (in total, about 2% of live births) will have a rise in unconjugated (indirect) bilirubin, whereas those with liver disease such as biliary atresia will have a rise in conjugated (direct) bilirubin.

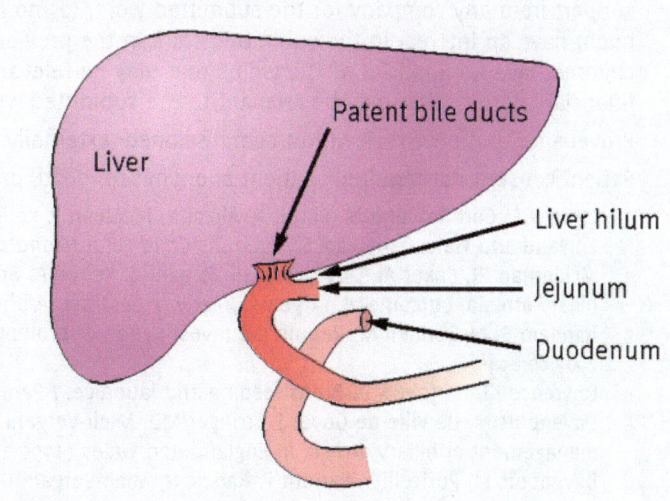

Fig 1 Kasai portoenterostomy with bowel attached to the liver hilum allowing unaffected patent bile ducts to drain into the intestine. Adapted from a line drawing supplied by Deirdre Kelly

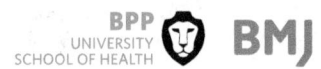

If the conjugated bilirubin is raised above normal (normal conjugated bilirubin <20 µmol/l) refer the infant to the local paediatric department for further liver function tests.

Refer all babies with suspected biliary atresia to a paediatric liver unit. A substantial rise in alkaline phosphatase and γ-glutamyltransferase, with a variable rise in alanine aminotransferase and aspartate aminotransferase, may suggest biliary atresia. The synthetic function of the liver (assessed by measuring albumin levels and prothrombin time) will be normal unless diagnosis is delayed, resulting in decompensated cirrhosis. Further testing in a specialist unit will include an ultrasound scan (showing a small gallbladder and hepatomegaly without biliary dilatation), a radionucleotide excretion scan or endoscopic retrograde cholangiopancreatography (confirming lack of flow of bile from the liver into the bowel), and a liver biopsy (showing biliary obstruction and fibrosis while excluding other conditions such as neonatal hepatitis). Intraoperative cholangiography is the definitive test for biliary atresia as it displays the abnormal biliary tree.[11]

How is it managed?

Children with biliary atresia initially need nutritional support with a high energy, high level, medium chain triglyceride feed such as Caprilon (SHS International) and oral supplementation with fat soluble vitamins (A, D E, and K) as biliary atresia impairs absorption of these vitamins.[11]

The Kasai portoenterostomy is usually performed at the same time as the intraoperative cholangiography and may restore the flow of bile (in 60% of cases) by removing the scarred proportion of the biliary tree and attaching a Roux-en-Y loop of bowel to the cut surface of the liver hilum so enabling small patent bile ducts to drain into the intestine (figure). Postoperative steroids are given to reduce inflammation and encourage bile flow. Postoperative complications include ascending cholangitis which is prevented by a rotating course of prophylactic antibiotics. Recurrent cholangitis is an indication for liver transplantation, and so prevention and prompt treatment is essential.[12] The presentation of ascending cholangitis is subtle but includes pyrexia, irritability, vomiting and abdominal pain with elevation of inflammatory markers and serum bilirubin.

All children should be followed up long term in a specialist liver centre so that complications (such as poor growth, vitamin deficiency, and the development of portal hypertension) and the need for liver transplantation can be monitored.

Contributors. All authors contributed equally to the preparation of this article.

Funding: No special funding.

Competing interests: All authors have completed the Unified Competing Interest form at www.icmje. org/coi_disclosure.pdf (available on request from the corresponding author) and declare (1) no support from any company for the submitted work; (2) no relationships with any companies that might have an interest in the submitted work in the previous 3 years; (3) their spouses, partners, or children have no financial relationships that may be relevant to the submitted work; and (4) no non-financial interests that may be relevant to the submitted work.

Provenance and peer review: Not commissioned; externally peer reviewed.

Patient consent not required (patient anonymised, dead, or hypothetical).

1 Livesey E, Cortina Borja M, Sharif K, Alizai N, McClean P, Kelly D, et al. Epidemiology of biliary atresia in England and Wales (1999-2006). *Arch Dis Child Fetal Neonatal Ed* 2009;94:F451-5.
2 McKiernan PJ, Baker AJ, Lloyd C, Mieli-Vergani G, Kelly DA. British paediatric surveillance unit study of biliary atresia: outcome at 13 years. *J Pediatr Gastroenterol Nutr* 2009;48(1):78-84.
3 Hannam S, McDonnell M, Rennie JM. Investigation of prolonged neonatal jaundice. *Acta Paediatrica* 2007;89:694-7.
4 Lawrence M, Gartner MD. Breastfeeding and jaundice. *J Perinatology* 2001;21:S25-9.
5 Davenport M, de Ville de Goyet J, Stringer MD, Mieli-Vergani G, Kelly DA, McClean P, et al. Seamless management of biliary atresia in England and Wales (1999-2002). *Lancet* 2004;363:1354-7.
6 Davenport M, Puricelli V, Farrant P, Hadzic N, Mieli-Vergani G, Portmann B, et al. The outcome of the older (> or =100 days) infant with biliary atresia. *J Pediatr Surg* 2004;39:575-81.
7 Serinet MO, Wildhaber BE, Broue P, Lachaux A, Sarles J, Jacquemin E, et al. Impact of age at Kasai operation on its results in late childhhod and adolescence: a rational basis for biliary atresia screening. *Pediatrics* 2009;123:1280-6.

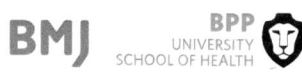

8 Davenport M, Tizzard SA, Underhill J, Mieli-Vergani G, Portmann B, Hadzic N. The biliary atresia splenic malformationsyndrome: a 28-year single-center retrospective study. *J Pediatr* 2006;149:393-400.

9 National Institute for Health and Clinical Excellence. Neonatal jaundice. (Clinical guideline 98.) 2010. www.nice.org.uk/CG98.

10 Crofts DJ, Michel VJ, Rigby AS, Tanner MS, Hall DM, Bonham JR. Assessment of stool colour in community management of prolonged jaundice in infancy. *Acta Paediatrica* 1999;88:969-74.

11 Hartley JL, Davenport M, Kelly DA. Biliary atresia. *Lancet* 2009;374:1704-13.

12 Shinkai M, Ohhama Y, Take H, Kitagawa N, Kudo H, Mochizuki K, et al. Long-term outcome of children with biliary atresia who were not transplanted after the Kasai operation: >20-years experience at a children's hospital. *J Pediatr Gastroenterol Nutr* 2009;48:443-50.

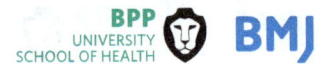

Congenital cataract

Heather C Russell, specialist registrar in ophthalmology[1],
Valerie McDougall, general practitioner[2], Gordon N Dutton, consultant
ophthalmologist[3]

[1]Princess Alexandra Eye
Pavilion, Edinburgh EH3
9HA, UK

[2]MacLean Medical
Practice, Glasgow G44
3QG, UK

[3]Royal Hospital for Sick
Children, Glasgow G3 8SJ

Correspondence to: H C
Russell heatherrussell74@
gmail.com

Cite this as: *BMJ*
2011;342:d3075

DOI: 10.1136/bmj.d3075

www.bmj.com/
content/342/bmj.d3075

Congenital cataract is an important preventable cause of visual impairment and blindness in childhood. Advances in surgical management and visual rehabilitation mean that early diagnosis is vital to optimise visual outcome and prevent irreversible visual impairment.

Why is congenital cataract missed?

In ideal conditions, examination for the red reflex by an experienced practitioner readily identifies congenital cataract; however, its effectiveness as a screening tool has yet to be formally evaluated. A national UK study assessing all diagnoses of congenital cataract during one year found that less than half were detected at either the newborn or 6-8 week examinations (35% at the newborn examination and a further 12% at the 6-8 week examination).[2] A more recent regional study from the Republic of Ireland found that over a 10 year period, none of the 27 cases of congenital cataract was detected at the neonatal check and only 24% were detected by the general practitioner on subsequent examination.[3] Although recommendations for red reflex detection as part of the newborn and 6-8 week examinations were in place at the time of these studies, no data were available on the percentage of infants who had such testing, so whether delays in diagnosis were caused by problems performing the test or by failure to test (assuming that most cataracts were present from birth) is unclear.[4][5]

Red reflex examination can be difficult to perform. Eyelid swelling at birth can make eye opening difficult, especially if the infant is distressed. Examination conditions can be suboptimal, with brightly lit rooms, background noise, and interruptions. Examination of infants aged 6-8 weeks is usually easier when eyelid swelling has resolved and they are more visually alert and maintain gaze.

Why does this matter?

Visually significant congenital cataracts lead to irreversible changes in the developing visual system owing to form-deprivation amblyopia, and they can also cause nystagmus. These disorders result in severe and lifelong visual impairment. Some evidence suggests that these changes start to develop after only 6 weeks of life for unilateral cataract and 10 weeks of life for bilateral cataracts.[6][7] Other evidence suggests that irreversible changes occur earlier,

---

KEY POINTS

- Congenital cataract is uncommon but is an important preventable cause of visual impairment and blindness
- For optimal visual outcome, surgical correction is needed within the first three months of birth as visual impairment may develop after only 6 weeks of life for unilateral cataract and after 10 weeks for bilateral cataracts
- In many countries, including the UK, ocular examination is recommended shortly after birth and again at 6-8 weeks
- Red reflex examination is used to detect opacities such as cataract, retinoblastoma, and malformations
- Red reflex examination needs optimal conditions, experience, and patience
- Detection of any abnormality warrants urgent ophthalmological referral

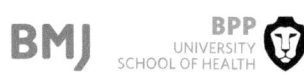
with long term visual outcomes showing an average loss of one Snellen visual acuity line for every three weeks of surgical delay during the first 14 weeks of life.[8] Cataract surgery is essential before these irreversible changes take place. Early detection is therefore vital.

How is congenital cataract diagnosed?

Screening for congenital cataract, other ocular media opacities, and ocular malformations requires the red reflex to be sought. Although recommendations for performance of this test shortly after birth and again at 6-8 weeks have been in place for many years,[4][5] red reflex examination has only recently achieved "screening programme" status as part of the National Screening Committee's NHS Newborn and Infant Physical Examination Programme (http://newbornphysical.screening.nhs.uk/).

During the test the room must be calm, quiet, and very dark. The infant is positioned comfortably on the mother's lap, with the head against her stomach. Calmly singing to the infant holds attention, often with spontaneous eye opening, and a bottle feed or soother can have the same effect. Alternatively, the infant can be positioned either over the mother's shoulder, or held head up at a 45° angle from the horizontal with one hand supporting the chest and the other hand used to jiggle the child's bottom (fig 1).[9] Both positions result in spontaneous eyelid opening. The largest white-light circle on the direct ophthalmoscope is used unless the pupils are very small, when the narrower light source is used. The lens is set at 0 or to the examiner's prescription if his or her glasses are removed. The examiner sits or stands at arm's length from the child and looks at the child's face through the aperture. If the infant is asleep, the eyelids can be gently opened with clean fingers. If the eyes are turned up (owing to Bell's phenomenon), the head can be turned gently from side to side to evoke the doll's eye phenomenon, which usually centres the eyes long enough to gain a view of the red reflex. Illumination of both pupils simultaneously is preferable to allow comparison. If a clear red reflex is not seen in one or both eyes, they are examined individually and compared.

Same day telephone referral to a paediatric ophthalmologist is warranted if the examination shows:

- The presence of opacities in the reflex (fig 2)
- The absence of any reflex
- A white pupillary reflex (leukocoria)

Urgent written referral to the ophthalmologist is recommended if the examination shows:

- Inequality in colour, intensity, or clarity of the reflection
- No detectable abnormality but a parent or observer describes a history suspicious of leukocoria on observation or in a photograph (recognising, however, that the commonest

---

CASE SCENARIO

A mother brings her 8 week old baby to her general practitioner for her 6-8 week child health surveillance check. At the baby's initial neonatal hospital check the doctor had difficulty performing the red reflex examination owing to neonatal eyelid swelling, but took no further action. The general practitioner cannot detect the red reflex in the right eye so makes a direct referral to the ophthalmologist that day by telephone. The baby is seen the following day and a cataract in the right eye is diagnosed. Cataract surgery is performed four days later.

HOW COMMON IS CONGENITAL CATARACT?

- In the United Kingdom the incidence of detected cataract of congenital origin affecting vision has been estimated to be 2.49 per 10000 population by age 1 year
- Owing to some delayed diagnoses, the incidence increases to 3.46 per 10000 population by age 15 years. This equates with 200-300 children being born with congenital cataract each year in the UK[1]

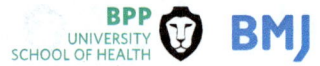

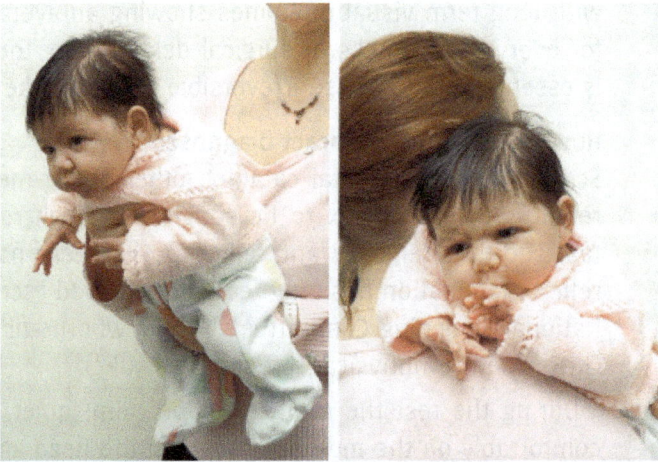

Fig 1 Positioning of an infant to induce spontaneous eye opening. Left: The child is held leaning forward at 45° to the horizontal, with one hand supporting the chest and the other supporting and jiggling the infant's bottom. Right: The child is positioned over the mother's shoulder

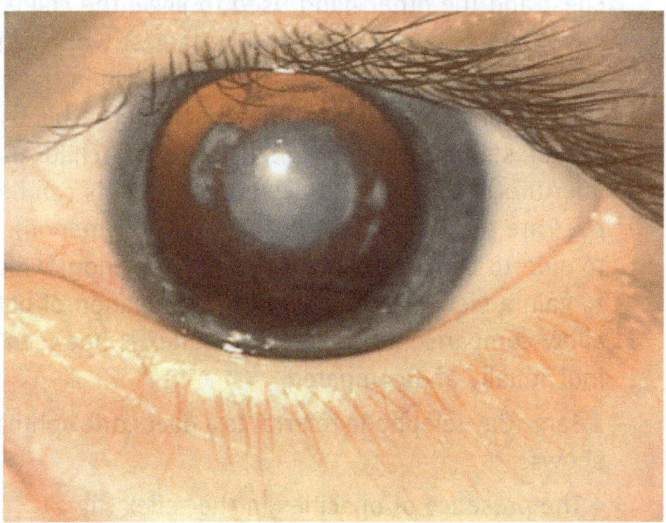

Fig 2 Red reflex showing a nuclear cataract

cause of a white pupil in flash photography is reflection from the optic disc of the in-turning eye when fixation is off-axis to the camera).[10]

In addition to the detection of media opacities, giving attention to eyes and vision at the time of the 6-8 week neonatal check has the potential to identify other conditions affecting sight, such as delayed visual maturation and nystagmus.

Screeners should be aware that the normal red reflex seen in dark skinned infants tends to be more yellow than red. This should not be confused with the white reflex of leukocoria, which may indicate underlying retinoblastoma.

Low specificity is expected to be the consequence of increasing the sensitivity of the red reflex test, leading to more false positive referrals. However, this is arguably acceptable in view of the serious and irreversible consequences of missed diagnoses.[11]

How is congenital cataract managed?
Visually significant congenital cataracts are managed by prompt cataract surgery, and the resulting aphakia is corrected with prolonged wear contact lenses, primary intraocular lens implantation, or aphakic spectacles. Long term follow-up with the ophthalmologist is needed.

Contributors: HCR contributed to the conception and design; to the acquisition and interpretation of data; and to the drafting and revising of the article. VMcD contributed to the conception and design; to the acquisition and interpretation of data; and to revising of the article critically for important

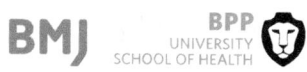

intellectual content. GND contributed to the conception and design and to revising of the article critically for important intellectual content. All authors approved the final version to be published. HCR and GND are the guarantors.

Competing interests: All authors have completed the Unified Competing Interest form at www.icmje. org/coi_disclosure.pdf (available on request from the corresponding author) and declare: no support from any organisation for the submitted work; no financial relationships with any organisations that might have an interest in the submitted work in the previous three years; no other relationships or activities that could appear to have influenced the submitted work.

Provenance and peer review: Commissioned; externally peer reviewed.

Patient consent obtained for the photos but not required for the case scenario (patient anonymised, dead, or hypothetical).

1   Rahi JS, Dezateux C. Measuring and interpreting the incidence of congenital ocular anomalies: lessons from a national study of congenital cataracts in the UK. *Invest Ophthalmol Vis Sci* 2001;42:1444-8.
2   Rahi JS, Dezateux C. National cross sectional study of detection of congenital and infantile cataract in the United Kingdom: role of childhood screening and surveillance. *BMJ* 1999;318:362-5.
3   Sotomi O, Ryan CA, O'Connor G, Murphy BP. Have we stopped looking for a red reflex in newborn screening? *Ir Med J* 2007;100:398-400.
4   Hall DM. Health for all children. 3rd ed. Report of the third joint working party on child health surveillance. Oxford University Press, 1996.
5   Royal College of Ophthalmologists, British Paediatric Association. Ophthalmic services for children. Report of joint working party. RCO, BPA, 1994.
6   Birch EE, Stager DR. The critical period for surgical treatment of dense congenital unilateral cataract. *Invest Ophthalmol Vis Sci* 1996;37:1532-8.
7   Lambert SR, Lynn MJ, Reeves R, Plager DA, Buckley EG, Wilson ME. Is there a latent period for the treatment of children with dense bilateral congenital cataracts? *JAAPOS* 2006;10:30-6.
8   Birch EE, Cheng C, Stager DR Jr, Weakley DR Jr, Stager DR Sr. The critical period for surgical treatment of dense congenital bilateral cataracts. *JAAPOS* 2009;13:67-71.
9   McLaughlin C, Levin AV. The red reflex. *Pediatric Emergency Care* 2006;22:137-40.
10 Russell HC, Agarwal PK, Somner JEA, Bowman RC, Dutton GN. Off-axis digital flash photography: a common cause of artefact leukocoria in children. *J Pediatr Ophthalmol Strabismus* 2010;46:e1-3.
11 Morgan S. In screening for congenital cataract, many false positive referrals will occur. *BMJ* 1999;319:122.

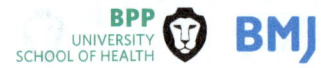

Hirschsprung's disease

A Arshad, paediatric specialist registrar[1],
C Powell, general practitioner[2],
M P Tighe, paediatric consultant[1]

[1]Paediatric Department, Poole Hospital NHS Trust, Poole BH15 2JB, UK

[2]Upton Surgery, Poole BH16 5PW

Correspondence to: Dr M P Tighe, Poole Hospital NHS Foundation Trust, Child Health, Poole Hospital, Longfleet Rd, Poole BH21 2HJ, UK
mpt195@hotmail.com

Cite this as: BMJ 2012;345:e5521

DOI: 10.1136/bmj.e5521

www.bmj.com/content/345/bmj.e5521

A 3 year old boy is brought to his general practitioner again by his worried mother. She is concerned that he remains constipated despite trying a third different laxative. Further history showed that he passed his first meconium only on day 5, and since then has been opening his bowels only weekly, with associated straining. His growth has fallen from the 25th to the 2nd centile for height and weight. On examination he has a distended abdomen with palpable stool throughout the abdomen.

What is Hirschsprung's disease?

Hirschsprung's disease is characterised by an absence of ganglion cells in the distal bowel, beginning at the internal sphincter and extending proximally. The resulting aganglionic segment of the colon fails to relax, causing a functional obstruction. Presentation is commonly in the first 28 days of life (neonatal period), with delayed passage of meconium and abdominal distension (see "Red flags" box). However, about 12% of patients present again in childhood with intractable constipation (not responsive to laxatives) and failure to thrive, with about a third of these presenting with enterocolitis.[1][2]

Why is Hirschsprung's disease missed?

Hirschsprung's disease mainly presents to primary care as delayed passage of meconium or as constipation.[2][9] Missed or delayed diagnoses are decreasing owing to vigilance in primary care and early biopsy, with the mean age at diagnosis falling from 18 months in the 1960s to 2.6 months in the past 10 years.[2][11] However, substantial numbers of children with Hirschsprung's disease still present late (after age 3 years). Many late presentations result from missed diagnoses in primary care, but delayed presentation to primary care is sometimes a contributing factor, particularly in developing countries.[9]

Guidelines from the National Institute for Health and Clinical Excellence (NICE) recommend that normal passage of meconium within 24 hours of birth should be confirmed at the newborn examination (within 72 hours of birth) and that the stooling pattern should be reviewed at the six week postnatal check by the general practitioner.[3] A retrospective review over five years of 429 Italian children who had had a rectal biopsy found that 47 had Hirschsprung's disease, of whom 10 (21%) had been referred from primary care after the age of 2 years, despite persistent symptoms since the neonatal period.[12] Another literature review found that 475 (97%) of 490 children with Hirschsprung's disease who presented after the age of 10 years (a rarer subgroup) had presented with symptoms that had persisted since the neonatal period—abdominal pain, distension, and constipation refractory to laxatives.[13]

However, some late presentations to primary care occur. For example, a retrospective Kuwaiti review found that 14 (14%) of 102 patients with confirmed Hirschsprung's disease were aged over 1 year at diagnosis.[10] The researchers attributed some of the delayed

---

KEY POINTS

- Consider Hirschsprung's disease in patients with delayed (>24 h) passage of meconium and in patients with intractable constipation with symptoms since the neonatal period
- Early diagnosis reduces mortality and morbidity (such as risk of stoma) and reduces risks from enterocolitis

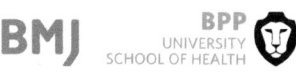

HOW COMMON IS HIRSCHSPRUNG'S DISEASE?

- 1 in 5000 live births a year[6]

- The male to female ratio is 4:1

- If the entire colon is involved, the sex ratio is about 1:1[5]

- With an affected sibling, the incidence rises to 12-33%[1][5]

- The prevalence is 1.5% in children with Down's syndrome[7]

- Over the past 20 years the proportion of delayed diagnoses in Hirschsprung's disease has fallen to a static level of 10-19%[2][8][9][10]

---

diagnoses to home laxative treatment and neglect of initial symptoms. And the Italian review cited above noted that 5% of children in their series had symptoms that started after the age of 1 year.[12]

Why does it matter?

Patients who have been referred late with Hirschsprung's disease may need more complicated corrective surgery, and older children with the disease have an increased risk of needing multiple operations and potentially a stoma, rather than the single stage pull-through operation for neonates.[2]

Delayed diagnosis of Hirschsprung's disease also increases the likelihood of associated enterocolitis, which is thought to arise from innately impaired colonic mucosal barrier against pathogens, an impairment that remains after surgery.[14] Patients present with shock, fever, and abdominal distension and may present as late as the age of 10 years and, less commonly, after surgical correction. Surgical correction for patients with enterocolitis associated with Hirschsprung's disease is more likely to necessitate a stoma. The Australian Paediatric Surveillance Unit found in 2003 that, among 127 children with Hirschsprung's disease, the incidence of associated enterocolitis was 33% (4/12 patients) in those with a late diagnosis, compared with only 12% (15/126) in those with a diagnosis in the neonatal period. The postoperative incidence of associated enterocolitis was 21% but with no deaths.[2] A rate of death from enterocolitis associated with Hirschsprung's disease of 5-25% in older series has now decreased to about 1% in more recent series.[2][15] This fall has been attributed to raised awareness in primary care, and earlier diagnosis.[2]

Unnecessary rectal biopsies in children with functional constipation can also be avoided with an appropriate history (see below). A 1998 UK retrospective review assessed the notes of 141 patients who had had a rectal biopsy, including 17 patients with Hirschsprung's disease. The researchers concluded that normal passage of meconium, and being symptom-

---

"RED FLAGS" FOR HIRSCHSPRUNG'S DISEASE*

- *Delayed (>24 h) meconium*—Present in 70-87% of cases of Hirschsprung's disease and in <1% of normal children[2][3]

- *Neonatal constipation*—Present in 90-95% of cases but in <7% of children with functional constipation[2][3]

- *Family history (affected sibling)*—Present in 12-33% of cases[4][5]

- *Poor growth*—Present in 25-30% of cases[2][3]

- *Abdominal distension*—Present in 76-85% of cases but in 20% of patients with functional constipation[2][3]

- *Down's syndrome and other chromosomal anomalies*—Hirschsprung's disease is present in 1.5% of patients with Down's syndrome, but 5-10% of patients with Down's have functional constipation[7]

*Three or more red flags are present in 18% of patients with the disease. No red flags are present in <1% of patients with the disease[2][3]

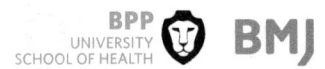

free beyond the age of 1 month, obviates the need for biopsy and that 60% of rectal biopsies performed to exclude Hirschsprung's disease would not have been indicated[4]; other studies, however, disagree with such a categorical statement.[3] [12]

How is Hirschsprung's disease diagnosed?

Clinical

The "Red flags" box lists features to look out for to avoid missing Hirschsprung's disease. Consider referring neonates with delayed passage of meconium (beyond 24 hours). Ninety five per cent of neonates with Hirschsprung's disease fail to pass meconium within the first 24 hours of life, compared with <1% of normal neonates.[8] [16] [17] Other common features include abdominal distension, a family history of Hirschsprung's disease, or other associated features.

Also refer older children with any of the features shown in the "Red flags" box. These features help to differentiate Hirschsprung's disease from functional constipation, which has an estimated prevalence of about 34% among preschool children in community surveys.[18] Only 5% of childhood constipation has an organic cause, and discussion of other causes can be found elsewhere.[19] Soiling is unlikely in Hirschsprung's disease.[11] In the UK retrospective review cited above,[4] 17 patients had Hirschsprung's disease and all had presented with symptoms within the first four weeks. Three of the 17 patients had been referred late (at ages 2 years, 11 months, and 3 years), and two had a positive family history.[20]

Features of Hirschsprung's disease on examination include failure to thrive, a distended abdomen, and explosive stools on digital rectal examination. The NICE guidelines on constipation advise that rectal examination should be performed only by healthcare professionals competent in recognising anorectal anatomical problems.[3] Rectal examination in the preceding 48 hours can potentially reduce the positive predictive value of barium enemas or anorectal manometry by decompressing the rectum.[21] NICE recommends urgent referral if Hirschsprung's disease is suspected clinically.[3]

Investigations

Hirschsprung's disease is diagnosed by identifying the absence of ganglion cells on rectal suction biopsy, which is generally taken about 2 cm above the dentate line of the rectum. Other investigations aim to reduce the number of referrals for rectal suction biopsies. These include anorectal manometry, barium enema, and plain abdominal radiography (figure), the last of which is useful in looking for any anomalies needing surgery in neonates with delayed passage of meconium and abdominal distension, and is readily available. A prospective study of 111 consecutive patients compared the relative sensitivities and specificities of these diagnostic tests for Hirschsprung's disease and found that anorectal manometry (83% sensitive, 93% specific) was similar to barium enema (76% sensitive, 93% specific), but rectal suction biopsy was superior (93% sensitive, 100% specific).[22]

How is Hirschsprung's disease managed?

The length of affected bowel can be variable, occasionally involving the whole colon, but generally restricted to the rectum and sigmoid.[8] Further management includes stabilisation (through resuscitation, antibiotics if indicated, and decompression, with a nasogastric tube and rectal washouts). This is followed by surgery, which allows identification and resection of the aganglionic section and, where possible, allows the normal ganglionic bowel to be brought down to be anastomosed to the anus in a single stage procedure while preserving sphincter function.[8]

Post-surgical morbidity has lessened with time. A case series in 2008 following 192 patients postoperatively showed no perioperative deaths but anastomotic leakage in four patients. At follow-up (at 6-40 months), of 145 patients, 7 had faecal incontinence, 8 had constipation, and 38 (26%) had had enterocolitis.[23] Enterocolitis is mainly managed conservatively, with intravenous fluids, bowel rest, and antibiotics.

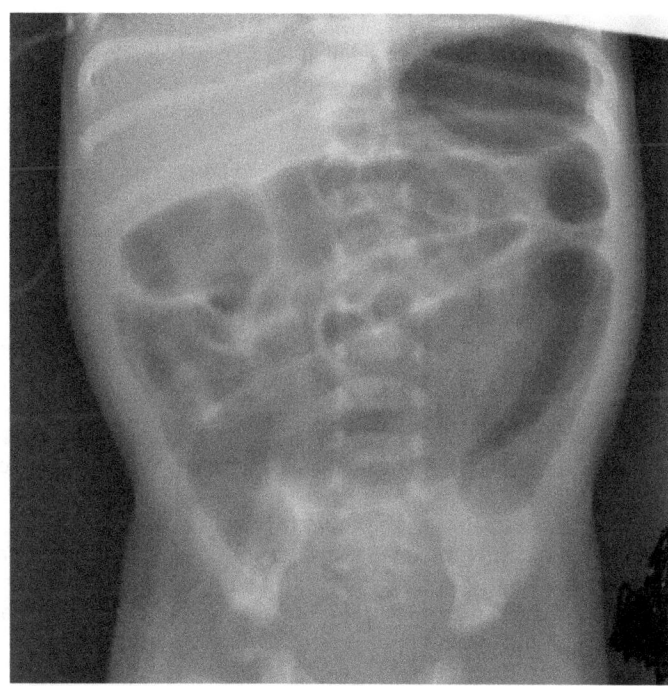

Fig 1 Abdominal x ray image showing gaseous distension of the large bowel with air absent from the rectum (typical of Hirschsprung's disease)

In the long term, most patients who have had Hirschsprung's disease enjoy an excellent quality of life, with near normal anorectal function after surgery, although some abnormalities of bowel function can persist.[14] One long term follow-up study found that 75-95% of patients achieve a stool frequency of <5 stools a day.[6] Parents should be advised of the increased risk of Hirschsprung's disease for any future children they have.[24]

Contributors: MPT conceived the article. AA did the literature search. All authors wrote the article, and MPT and CP edited it. MPT is the guarantor.

Competing interests: All authors have completed the ICMJE uniform disclosure form at www.icmje. org/coi_disclosure.pdf (available on request from the corresponding author) and declare: no support from any organisation for the submitted work; no financial relationships with any organisations that might have an interest in the submitted work in the previous three years; no other relationships or activities that could appear to have influenced the submitted work.

Provenance and peer review: Not commissioned; externally peer reviewed.

Consent obtained from the parents for publication of both the case history and the abdominal x ray image.

1   Kleinhaus S, Boley SJ, Sheran M, Sieber WK. Hirschsprung's disease—a survey of the members of the surgical section of the American Academy of Pediatrics. *J Pediatr Surg* 1979;14:588.
2   Singh SJ, Croaker GDH, Manglick P, Wong CLH, Athanasakos H, Elliott E, et al. Hirschsprung's disease: the Australian Paediatric Surveillance Unit's experience. *Ped Surg Int* 2003;19:247-50.
3   National Institute for Health and Clinical Excellence. Diagnosis and management of idiopathic childhood constipation in primary and secondary care. (Clinical guidance 99.) 2010. http://guidance.nice.org.uk/CG99.
4   Ghosh A, Griffiths DM. Rectal biopsy in the investigation of constipation. *Arch Dis Child* 1998;79:266-8.
5   Suita S, Taguchi T, Ieiri S, Nakatsuji T. Hirschsprung's disease in Japan: analysis of 3852 patients based on a nationwide survey in 30 years. *J Pediatr Surg* 2005;40:197.
6   Hackam DJ, Filler RM, Pearl RH. Enterocolitis after the surgical treatment of Hirschsprung's disease: risk factors and financial impact. *J Pediatr Surg* 1998;33:830.
7   Torfs C, Christianson RE. Anomalies in Down syndrome individuals in a large population-based registry. *Am J Med Genet* 1999;77:431-8.
8   Haricharan RN, Seo J-M, Kelly DR, Mroczek-Musulman EC, Aprahamian CJ, Morgan TL, et al. Older age at diagnosis of Hirschsprung disease decreases risk of postoperative enterocolitis, but resection of additional ganglionated bowel does not. *J Ped Surg* 2008;43:6:1115-23.
9   Nofech-Mozes Y, Rachmel A, Schonfeld T, Schwarz M, Steinberg R, Ashkenazi S. Difficulties in making the diagnosis of Hirschsprung disease in early infancy. *J Paediatr Child Health* 2004;40:716-9.
10 Ziad F, Katchy KC, Al Ramadan S, Alexander S, Kumar S. Clinicopathological features in 102 cases of Hirschsprung disease. *Ann Saudi Med* 2006;26:200-4.
11 Rescorla FJ, Morrison AM, Engles D, West KW, Grosfeld JL. Hirschsprung's disease: evaluation of mortality and long-term function in 260 cases. *Arch Surg* 1992;127:934-41.

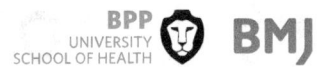

12 Pini-Prato A, Avanzini S, Gentilino V, Martucciello G, Mattioli G, Coccia C, et al. Rectal suction biopsy in the workup of childhood chronic constipation: indications and diagnostic value. *Pediatr Surg Int* 2007;23:117-22.

13 Doodnath R, Puri P. A systematic review and meta-analysis of HD presenting after childhood. *Ped Surg Int* 2010;26:1107-10.

14 Aslam A, Spicer RD, Corfield AP. Children with Hirschsprung's disease have an abnormal colonic mucus defensive barrier independent of the bowel innervation status. *J Pediatr Surg* 1997;32:1206-10.

15 Ikeda K, Goto S. Diagnosis and treatment of Hirschsprung's disease in Japan: an analysis of 1628 patients. *Ann Surg* 1984;199:400-5.

16 Sherry SN, Kramer I. The time of passage of the first stool and first urine by a newborn infant. *J Pediatr* 1955;46:158.

17 Clark DA. Times of first void and first stool in 500 newborns. *Pediatrics* 1977;60:457.

18 Swenson O, Sherman JO, Fisher JH. Diagnosis of congenital megacolon: an analysis of 501 patients. *J Pediatr Surg* 1973;8:587.

19 Afzal NA, Tighe MP, Thomson MA. Constipation in children: a review. *Ital J Ped* 2011;37:28.

20 Teitelbaum DH, Qualman SJ, Caniano DA. Hirschsprung's disease. Identification of risk factors for enterocolitis. *Ann Surg* 1988;207:240-4.

21 Blake NS. Diagnosis of Hirschsprung's disease and allied disorders. In: Holschneider AM, Puri P, eds. Hirschsprung's disease and allied disorders. Harwood Academic Publishers, 2010:223-90.

22 De Lorijn F, Reitsma JB, Voskuijl WP, Aronson DC, ten Kate FJ, Smets AM, et al. Diagnosis of Hirschsprung's disease: a prospective, comparative accuracy study of common tests. *J Pediatrics* 2005;146:787-92.

23 Liem NT, Hau BD. One-stage operation for Hirschsprung's disease: experience with 192 cases. *Asian J Surg* 2008;31:216-9.

24 Chakravarti A, Lyonnet S. Hirschsprung disease. In: Scriver CR, Beaudet AR, Sly W, Valle D, eds. The metabolic and molecular bases of inherited disease. 8th ed. McGraw-Hill, 2001.

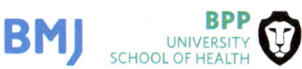

Streptococcal perianal infection in children

Richard Lehman, general practitioner[1],
Sarah Pinder, general practitioner[1]

[1]Hightown Surgery,
Banbury OX16 9DB

Correspondence to: R
Lehman richard.lehman@
nhs.net

Cite this as: *BMJ*
2009;338:b1517

DOI: 10.1136/bmj.b1517

www.bmj.com/
content/338/bmj.b1517

Streptococcal perianal infection in children is caused by group A *Streptococcus pyogenes* and is usually confined to the immediate perianal area, though it can spread to the perineum and occasionally the genitalia.[1][2]

How common is it?

The incidence of perianal infection caused by group A *S pyogenes* is not known, but since the first case descriptions in 1966[3] it has been reported in children from around the world. In a US general paediatric practice, perianal streptococcal disease was detected in one consultation per 300, and perineal disease (that is, perianal plus vulvovaginal disease) in one per 200.[1] A 1996 audit of our own practice (an urban British practice with 7000 patients and four full time general practitioners), found that 18 cases had been detected over two years by general practitioners highly aware of the condition—about one consultation per 1000 patients (children and adults combined). On this basis, the average general practitioner in the United Kingdom might expect to see childhood streptococcal perianal disease once or twice a year. It occurs in prepubertal children from infancy, with a peak incidence between the ages of 3 and 5 years.[4]

Why is it missed?

We conducted a postal survey of all general practitioners in north Oxfordshire in 1996 (table) using the presentation from the case scenario in this article. The findings showed that most respondents were not aware of streptococcal disease as a likely diagnosis despite a classic presentation with pain on defecation, erythema, and multiple fissures. The choice of treatments suggests that likely diagnoses were thought to be threadworm infestation, simple constipation, or fungal infection, with nine of the 54 respondents mentioning the possibility of sexual abuse. There is, however, no clear evidence that perianal redness and fissures should in themselves be taken as indicators of possible sexual abuse.[5] The main reason that paediatric streptococcal perianal infection is missed in primary care may be lack of awareness.

Why does this matter?

The natural course of untreated perianal streptococcal infection in children is not known, but it is known that it can cause prolonged discomfort, toilet avoidance, and constipation,[1] [4][6] and given the findings of our 1996 survey we think it might raise unfounded suspicion of child abuse. From our survey and from several case series reports, it seems likely that inappropriate initial treatment is common. Infection can spread to siblings and other

---

KEY POINTS

- Bright red perianal rash in preschool children, especially with fissuring, is often caused by streptococcal infection
- Most general practitioners will see one or two cases a year
- The diagnosis is established by a pure growth of group A streptococcus from a perianal swab
- Treatment is with co-amoxiclav or clarithromycin for 7-10 days

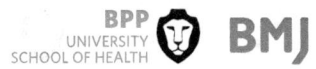

Table 1 Responses of 54 (68% response rate)* general practitioners in north Oxfordshire to the case presented in the scenario cited in this article when asked: "What would be your management at this first consultation?"

Suggested management	No (%) of general practitioners
Treat with anthelmintics	29 (54)
Treat with antifungal cream	12 (22)
Treat with topical anaesthetics	15 (28)
Treat with topical antiseptics	6 (11)
Take a perianal swab	17 (31)
Treat with stool softeners	28 (52)
Treat with systemic antibiotics	4 (7)

"Free text" responses (outside the options suggested in the questionnaire) included looking for possible sexual abuse (9; 17%) and looking for inflammatory bowel disease (4; 7%).
*Questionnaires were sent to 80 general practitioners.

CASE SCENARIO

A 3 year old child is brought by her mother, who says that her daughter has had an itchy bottom and pain on opening her bowels most days for the past two weeks. On examination she has an erythematous and excoriated anus with multiple anal fissures. As these symptoms and findings in a preschool child are highly suggestive of streptococcal proctitis, you undertake a perianal swab, which shows a pure growth of group A streptococcus.

---

children[7] and inadequate treatment may be followed by recurrence. Complications include local tissue spread and, less commonly, an illness similar to scarlet fever (guttate psoriasis) and glomerulonephritis.

How is it diagnosed?

Clinical features

Several case series describe the clinical features of perianal streptococcal infection,[1 4 6] although variations in reporting make it difficult to specify the exact prevalence or the predictive value against the optimal bacteriological proof:

- Constipation: about half of cases

- Pain on defecation of recent onset: about half of cases

- Itching: a quarter of cases in one series[8] and 78% and 100% in others

- Blood seen in stools: 20-35%

- Erythema: over 90% in most case series, although this is also common in asymptomatic children (41% in a descriptive study of 267 prebubertal, non-abused children[4]). The erythema is often described as bright or "beefy" (figure). A distinct margin may be commoner in streptococcal infection

- Fissures: about a quarter in one series,[9] absent in the normal child population[5]

- Exudate and/or visible bleeding on examination: sometimes mentioned.

Investigations

Definitive diagnosis is by the growth of a pure culture of group A streptococcus from a perianal swab. External anal examination and gentle perianal swabbing should therefore be performed whenever a child presents with clinical features suggestive of this infection. Such examination does not cause distress in the great majority of non-abused preschool children.[10]

How is it treated?

Observational evidence suggests a better response to treatment with oral co-amoxiclav or clarithromycin for 7-10 days than with oral phenoxymethylpenicillin (penicillin V).[4] The place of topical treatment is uncertain.

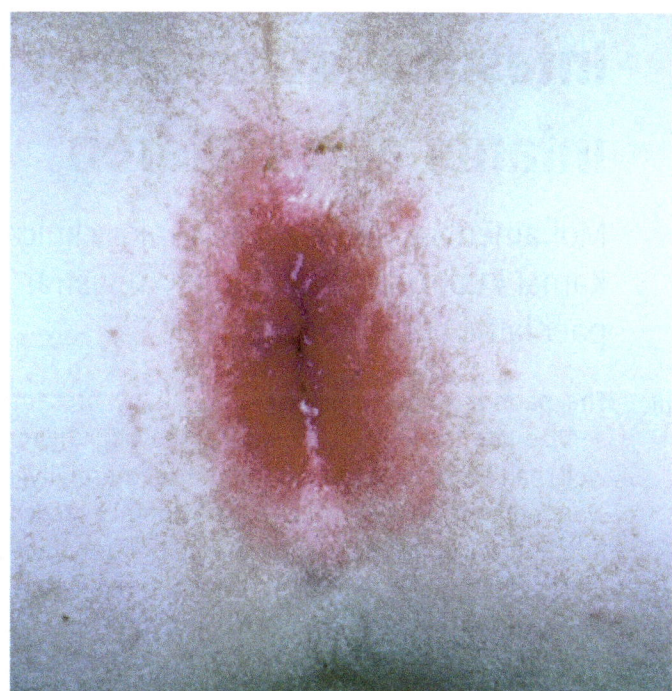

Fig 1 Streptococcal proctitis in child showing fissures and vivid red erythema ("raw beef") with a demarcated edge

Maureen Rogers provided the image of streptococcal proctitis.

Competing interests: None declared.

Contributors: SP carried out the survey mentioned in the text, and both authors did the literature searches and contributed to the preparation and editing of the manuscript. RL is the guarantor.

Provenance and peer review: Commissioned; externally peer reviewed.

Patient consent not required (patient anonymised, dead, or hypothetical).

1 Moglielnicki NP, Schwartzman JD, Elliott JA. Perineal group A streptococcal disease in a pedatric practice. *Pediatrics* 2000;106:276-81.
2 Kyriazi NC, Costenbader CL. Group A beta-hemolytic streptococcal balanitis: it may be more common than you think. *Pediatrics* 1991;88:154-6.
3 Amren DP, Anderson AS, Wannamaker LW. Perianal cellulitis associated with group A streptococcus. *Am J Dis Child* 1966;112:546.
4 Kokx NP, Comstock JA, Facklam RR. Streptococcal perianal disease in children. *Pediatrics* 1987;80:659-63.
5 McCann J, Voris J, Simon M, Wells R. Perianal findings in prepubertal children selected for nonabuse: a descriptive study. *Child Abuse Negl* 1989;13:179-93.
6 Wright JE, Butt HL. Perianal infection with beta haemolytic streptocoocus. *Arch Dis Child* 1994;70:145-6.
7 Petersen JP, Kaltoft MS, Misfeldt JC, Schumacher H, Schønheyder HC. Community outbreak of perianal group A streptococcal infection in Denmark. *Pediatr Infect Dis J* 2003;22:105-9.
8 Landolt M, Heininger U. Prevalence of perianal streptococcal dermatitis in children and adolescents. *Schweiz Rundsch Med Prax* 2005;94:1467-71.
9 Echeverria FM, Lopez-Menchero OJ, Maranon PR, Miguez NC, Sanchez SC, Vasquez LP. Isolation of group A hemolytic streptococcus in children with perianal dermatitis. *An Pediatr (Barc)* 2006;64:153-7.
10 Gulla K, Fenheim GE, Myhre AK, Lydersen S. Non-abused preschool children's perception of an anogenital examination. *Child Abuse Negl* 2007;31:885-94.

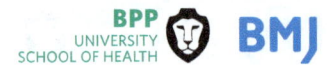

Intestinal malrotation and volvulus in infants and children

Mohamed Sameh Shalaby, senior clinical fellow in paediatric surgery, Kamal Kuti, paediatric surgery registrar, Gregor Walker, consultant paediatric surgeon

Department of Paediatric Surgery, Royal Hospital for Sick Children, Glasgow, UK

Correspondence to: M S Shalaby mshalaby@ doctors.org.uk

Cite this as: *BMJ* 2013;347:f6949

DOI: 10.1136/bmj.f6949

www.bmj.com/ content/347/bmj.f6949

The parents of a 2 week old term baby presented to the out of hours general practice service late in the evening with a two hour history of green vomiting. As the baby looked well, had been passing stools and urine normally, and had a soft non-tender abdomen, they were advised to attend their own general practice the following morning. The baby arrived in the local emergency department by ambulance six hours later with intractable shock. After aggressive resuscitation, the baby was taken to theatre for emergency laparotomy that revealed intestinal ischaemia from midgut volvulus associated with malrotation.

What is intestinal malrotation and volvulus?

Intestinal malrotation occurs because of failure of the normal sequence of rotation and fixation of the bowel (fig 1). Duodenal obstruction can occur due to extrinsic compression from bands leading from the caecum to the lateral abdominal wall (Ladd's bands) or from small bowel volvulus, which also leads to ischaemia of the midgut from superior mesenteric artery occlusion (fig 2).[1] Midgut volvulus can lead to irreversible intestinal necrosis, which is potentially fatal.[1]

Why is it missed?

Up to 80% of patients present in the first month of life,[2] and in this age group the cardinal symptom is bile (green) vomiting due to duodenal obstruction through midgut volvulus.[3] In a retrospective audit of 60 children presenting with malrotation or volvulus as an emergency to the Royal Hospital for Sick Children, Glasgow, over 13 years (1998-2010), 39 patients were less than 1 month old. In this group, despite green vomiting being present in 97%, 28 patients (72%) had symptoms for more than 24 hours before referral, and 32 patients (82%) had midgut volvulus at emergency laparotomy. In our experience, most of these patients have prior contact with community or hospital healthcare professionals that could result in earlier referral, which was also highlighted in a recently published case report.[4] Questionnaire surveys show that parents, midwifery staff, and other healthcare professionals may not appreciate the potential importance of true green vomit.[5] [6]

Up to 20% of patients with malrotation present after the first year of life,[1] and among these acute presentation with volvulus is less common. In the above mentioned 13 year institutional audit of children presenting with malrotation or volvulus as an emergency, 12 patients were more than 1 year old. Of these, only five patients (42%) had produced green coloured vomit at presentation and only three (25%) had midgut volvulus at emergency laparotomy. In this age group, lack of awareness and the development of more chronic,

---

KEY POINTS

- Green coloured vomit should prompt urgent surgical consultation even in an otherwise well child, as this may represent midgut volvulus
- Refer or investigate children with chronic unexplained abdominal symptoms to exclude rotational abnormalities
- Upper gastrointestinal contrast study is the investigation of choice
- Urgent surgical intervention is the key to avoid serious morbidity and mortality

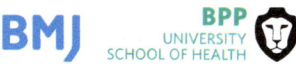

HOW COMMON IS INTESTINAL MALROTATION?

- The incidence of intestinal malrotation is about 1 in 500 live births, though autopsy studies estimate that it may be as high as 1% of the total population[2]

- The prevalence of volvulus is difficult to quantify, but any patient with malrotation is considered at a risk of midgut volvulus

- Despite the critical nature of this condition and the need for prompt surgical correction, many reports show delay between the onset of symptoms and surgical intervention[2 3 4]

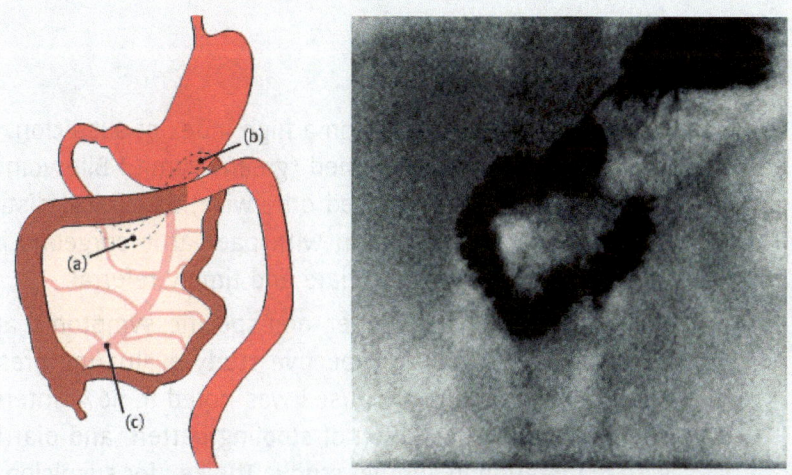

Fig 1 Left: Diagram of normal intestinal rotation. The third part of the duodenum (a) should cross the midline, with the fourth part (b) ascending on the left of the midline to the same level as the pylorus. Shaded part of bowel represents the midgut that is exclusively supplied by the superior mesenteric artery (c). Right: Normal upper gastrointestinal contrast study

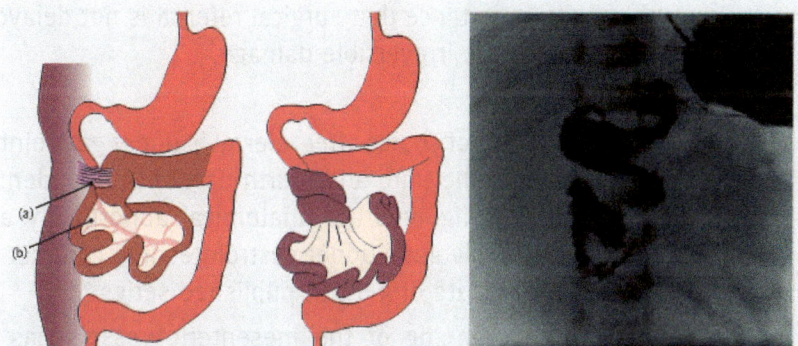

Fig 2 Left: Diagram of classic intestinal malrotation with abnormal duodenal fixation, Ladd's bands crossing the duodenum (a), and narrow base of mesentery (b). Centre: Diagram of small bowel volvulus with secondary ischaemia of the midgut. Right: Upper gastrointestinal contrast study of volvulus showing the characteristic "corkscrew" appearance

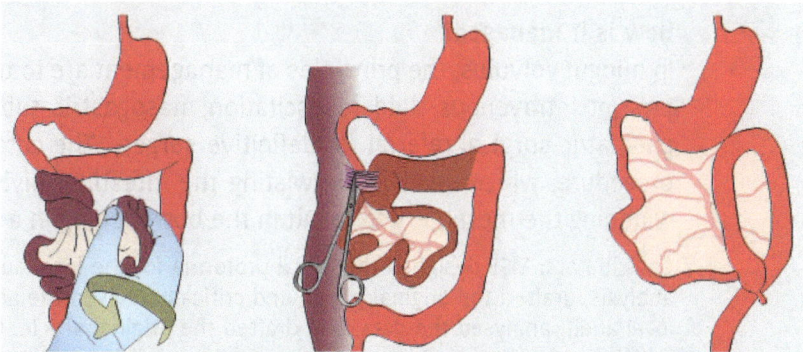

Fig 3 Operative steps of Ladd's procedure for small bowel volvulus, denoting (left) untwisting the intestine, (centre) dividing any adhesive bands, and (right) widening the mesentery to result in the bowel being in a "safe" non-rotated position

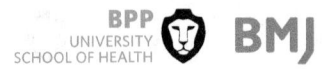

non-specific symptoms may make the diagnosis of malrotation difficult, particularly if the patient is already mislabelled as having "abdominal migraine or psychogenic pain or cyclic vomiting."[1] [3]

Why does it matter?

Midgut volvulus results in intestinal ischaemia, which may progress, until definitive surgery is undertaken to derotate the bowel. Delay in the diagnosis can lead to intestinal infarction with a substantial risk of mortality and morbidity including sepsis, short bowel syndrome, and the need for long term parenteral nutrition.[6]

How is it diagnosed?

Clinical

Clinical diagnosis is based on a high index of suspicion. Most neonates with malrotation or volvulus will have bile stained (green) vomit.[3] Bile vomiting should be considered to have a surgical cause until proved otherwise, as clinical distinction from non-surgical causes is difficult.[7] Prompt discussion with paediatric surgeons is advised in any baby with green vomiting to ensure appropriate and timely referral.

Pain, irritability, and other non-specific symptoms are more common in toddlers and older children.[2] In a retrospective study evaluating presentations of intestinal malrotation in children, anorexia or nausea was noted in 36%, intermittent apnoea in 24%, and failure to thrive in 41%.[3] Variation of stooling pattern and diarrhoea was noted in 16% of patients with malrotation in another study.[1] The key for suspicion and referral in the older patients is recurrent episodes of unexplained abdominal pain, irritability, vomiting, or failure to thrive.

Although late signs of volvulus include peritonitis, rectal bleeding, and end stage hypovolaemic shock, the lack of early signs can be falsely reassuring, with abdominal examination remaining unremarkable until intestinal ischaemia is advanced. It is of paramount importance that surgical referral is not delayed until the onset of those signs as they may indicate irreversible damage.

Investigations

The investigation of choice after referral is upper gastrointestinal contrast study to assess the configuration of the third and fourth part of the duodenum.[1] Figure 1 illustrates the normal duodenum, and figure 2 the anatomical abnormality and the characteristic "corkscrew" appearance in volvulus.[8] Upper gastrointestinal contrast study had a sensitivity of 96% and a false negative rate of 3-6% in published series.[9]

Ultrasound scanning of the mesenteric vessels has been suggested as a reasonable alternative, with reported sensitivity of 86.5%, specificity of 75%, positive predictive value of 42%, and negative predictive value of 96%.[10] We do not routinely use ultrasonography in the diagnosis, but it may be a useful adjunctive to assess the peristalsis and vascularity of the bowel in equivocal cases.

How is it managed?

In midgut volvulus, the principles of management are to treat haemodynamic instability with prompt intravenous fluid resuscitation, nasogastric tube decompression, and immediate paediatric surgical referral for definitive surgery. The curative surgical treatment is a Ladd's procedure, which involves untwisting the intestine, division of any congenital bands, and widening the mesentery to result in the bowel being in a "safe" non-rotated position (fig 3).

Contributors: MSS designed the initial proforma for the local audit, supervised the audit data analysis, drafted the original paper, and critically revised the article. KK collected the data from the local audit, analysed the data, and drafted the original article. GW supervised and helped with the initial data analysis and interpretation, and critically revised the article. All authors finally approved the published version.

Competing interests: We have read and understood the BMJ Group policy on declaration of interests and have no relevant interests to declare.

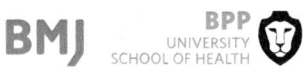

Provenance and peer review: Not commissioned; externally peer reviewed.

1   Millar AJW, Rode H, Cywes S. Malrotation and volvulus in infancy and childhood. *Semin Pediatr Surg* 2003;12:229-36.

2   Durkin ET, Lund DP, Shaaban AF, Schurr MJ, Weber SM. Age-related differences in diagnosis and morbidity of intestinal malrotation. *J Am Coll Surg* 2008;206:658-63.

3   Powell DM, Othersen HB, Smith CD. Malrotation of the intestines in children: the effect of age on presentation and therapy. *J Pediatr Surg* 1989;124:777-80.

4   Radwan R, Ram AD, Huddart SN. A few hours from disaster. *BMJ* 2012;345:e4441.

5   Walker GM, Neilson A, Young D, Raine PA. Colour of bile vomiting in intestinal obstruction in the newborn: questionnaire study. *BMJ* 2006;332:1363.

6   Walker GM, Raine PA. Bilious vomiting in the newborn: how often is further investigation undertaken? *J Pediatr Surg* 2007;42:714-6.

7   Millar AJW, Rode H, Brown RA, Cywes S. The deadly vomit: malrotation and midgut volvulus. *Pediatr Surg Int* 1987;2:172-6.

8   Sizemore AW, Rabbani KZ, Ladd A, Applegate KE. Diagnostic performance of the upper gastrointestinal series in the evaluation of children with clinically suspected malrotation. *Pediatr Radiol* 2008;38:518-28

9   Applegate KE. Evidence-based diagnosis of malrotation and volvulus. *Pediatr Radiol* 2009;39(suppl 2):S161-3.

10 Orzech N, Navarro OM, Langer JC. Is ultrasonography a good screening test for intestinal malrotation? *J Pediatr Surg* 2006;41:1005-9.

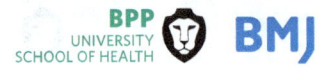

Cow's milk allergy in children

John R Apps, foundation year 1, academic foundation programme[1],
R Mark Beattie, consultant paediatric gastroenterologist[2]

[1]North Central Thames
Foundation School
Barnet and Chase Farm
NHS Trust, Enfield,
London EN2 8JL

[2]Paediatric Medical Unit,
Southampton General
Hospital, Southampton
SO16 6YD

Correspondence to: R M
Beattie Mark.beattie@
suht.swest.nhs.uk

Cite this as: BMJ
2009;339:b2275

DOI: 10.1136/bmj.b2275

http://www.bmj.com/
content/339/bmj.b2275

Cow's milk (protein) allergy is an adverse immunological response to cow's milk proteins seen mainly in the first few years of life. It can have diverse manifestations. It can be broadly divided into IgE (type I hypersensitivity) mediated disease and non-IgE (usually type IV hypersensitivity) mediated disease, sometimes referred to as cow's milk (protein) intolerance. These differ in clinical presentation, diagnostic testing, and prognosis; for example, type I hypersensitivity classically presents early, with symptoms such as urticaria, wheeze, and vomiting; non-IgE mediated symptoms are often delayed and protean, although most affect the skin and gastrointestinal systems. However, the two conditions overlap.

Why is it missed?

In a large prospective birth cohort study of 2138 families that investigated cow's milk allergy and egg allergy, more than a third of children with confirmed reactions were not on appropriate dietary restriction.[5] Only 54% of the parents of the 206 children with perceived allergy (by the parents) discussed it with their doctor, and a fifth of parentally initiated restriction diets were inappropriate.[5] Engagement with medical services was lacking; this, together with the diverse and potentially multifactorial aetiologies of presentations and the varied diagnostic pathways, probably resulted in underdiagnosis.

Why does this matter?

Cow's milk allergy can have several severe manifestations, either directly or indirectly through inappropriate management. Inappropriate dietary restriction independent of adequate medical and dietary supervision can cause morbidity in the infant or mother (or both), through inadequate intake of dietary components, especially calcium.[6] In extreme cases this can lead to rickets.[6] Acutely, IgE mediated cow's milk allergy can result in anaphylaxis, hypoxia, and shock. Chronically, either form can lead to anaemia, hypoalbuminaemia, and faltering growth.

Accurate diagnosis and engagement of families is therefore necessary for optimum outcome in children with confirmed or parentally perceived cow's milk allergy. Failure of this can cause families to resort to medical or paramedical practitioners who offer non-validated tests and inadequately supervised treatment regimens.

How is it diagnosed?

Clinical features

Cow's milk allergy encompasses a wide range of clinical manifestations, from the relatively benign to those that are life threatening. Symptoms usually begin within the first month of life, or within a week after introduction of cow's milk formula. More than one body system is usually affected—often the skin (50-70%; urticaria or atopic dermatitis), gastrointestinal tract (50-60%; nausea, vomiting, diarrhoea, or colic), and respiratory system (20-30%; rhinoconjunctivitis or wheeze).[1] Box 1 lists features that are suggestive of a diagnosis of cow's milk allergy. Infants without classic early onset symptoms of type I hypersensitivity (urticaria, wheeze, vomiting, and irritability) either present with a range of symptoms within hours to days of ingestion, such as in case 2, or present with common infant ailments (box 2). Unlike infants with type I hypersensitivity reactions, these infants are often IgE negative. They are harder to recognise, and children who present with complex symptoms of unclear aetiology should be considered for specialist referral.

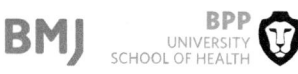

HOW COMMON IS IT?

- Large birth cohort studies that used elimination and challenge testing have shown that cow's milk allergy affects 2-3% of children,[1] and 0.5% of purely breastfed infants[1]

- It is the most common food allergy in infants and the most common cause of death from food related anaphylaxis in children in the United Kingdom[2][3]

- Estimates suggest that immediate type I hypersensitivity reactions, such as in case 1, occur in only 27-58% of cases[4]

BOX 1 FACTORS SUGGESTIVE OF COW'S MILK ALLERGY[1][7][8]

- Temporal association between symptoms and the ingestion of milk

- Several body systems affected. Most commonly the skin, gastrointestinal tract, and respiratory system, particularly if symptoms of atopic diseases are present (such as atopic dermatitis or asthma)

- Presence of a family history of atopy

- Exclusion of lactose intolerance, which manifests as explosive watery diarrhoea after ingestion of cow's milk

- Positive allergy tests or indicators of inflammation—for example, skin prick tests, specific IgE testing, eosinophilia on blood count

- Failure to respond to other treatments, including consideration of functional causes

BOX 2 COMMON INFANT PRESENTATIONS AND COW'S MILK ALLERGY

Atopic dermatitis
The National Institute for Health and Clinical Excellence recommends that food allergy should be considered in patients who have previously reacted to foods, or have moderate or severe disease not controlled on optimum management, particularly if associated with other symptoms of food allergy or faltering growth.[9]

Infantile colic
Two systematic reviews have supported the use of hypoallergenic formulas to reduce symptoms in infantile colic. However, methodological concerns have been expressed, and because of the benign, probably multifactorial, and self limiting nature of colic, the clinical importance of this finding remains uncertain.[10][11]

Gastro-oesophageal reflux and cow's milk allergy
Elimination and challenge testing have shown a clear overlap between gastro-oesophageal reflux and cow's milk allergy. A trial of cow's milk elimination could be considered in infants with other features of atopy or those who fail to respond to pharmacological management of their reflux.[12]

Other gastrointestinal symptoms
Cow's milk allergy should be considered in acute and chronic gastrointestinal presentations. It is associated with several gastrointestinal syndromes, including dietary protein induced proctitis (mild diarrhoea and rectal bleeding), dietary protein enteropathy and enterocolitis (vomiting, chronic diarrhoea, malabsorption, and failure to thrive with or without inflammation), and eosinophilic gastroenteropathies.[8]

Diagnostic testing
The diagnosis of cow's milk allergy is based on complete dietary elimination and challenge. In infants who are exclusively breast fed, cow's milk must be completely eliminated from the mother's diet. After elimination, the diagnosis should be confirmed by challenge, which should be performed under specialist guidance. In infants who are at risk of, or who have

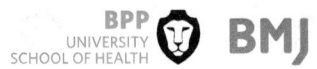

> **CASE SCENARIOS**
>
> *Case 1*
>
> A 3 month old infant, previously breast fed, presented with a urticarial rash, irritability, and vomiting shortly after introduction of cow's milk formula. He was referred to a paediatric allergy clinic where skin prick testing and specific IgE testing were positive for cow's milk protein. The mother did not wish to continue breast feeding. The formula was changed to an extensively hydrolysed protein feed, and the symptoms resolved rapidly. Re-challenge with cow's milk was deferred until 12 months and proceeded uneventfully.
>
> *Case 2*
>
> An otherwise well and thriving 6 week old breast fed infant presented with frequent stools, irritability, and perianal redness. Because physical examination was otherwise unremarkable and stool virology and culture were negative, he was referred to the paediatric (gastroenterology) outpatients department. Dietary protein induced proctocolitis was suspected. Because cow's milk is the most common allergen implicated in this condition, the mother was advised to stop taking all dairy products, but to continue breast feeding. The symptoms resolved within 72 hours but reappeared on challenge. The mother therefore continued to avoid dairy products while breast feeding (an extensively hydrolysed feed would be an alternative), and the infant was weaned at 6 months on to dairy free solids. Cow's milk was reintroduced at 12 months, and the child's original symptoms did not recur. The mother was referred for dietetic advice and prescribed calcium supplements.

a history of, severe reactions (previous severe reaction, positive specific IgE test, coexisting asthma, or enterocolitis), this should occur in hospital with adequate resuscitation support.[7]

In patients with a history compatible with type I hypersensitivity, specific IgE testing (previously known as IgE RAST testing) or referral to specialists for skin prick testing is useful (specific IgE testing: positive predictive testing, 90-95%; skin prick testing, negative predictive testing >95%, positive predictive testing <50%).[3] [7] [13] This may allow delay of challenges until likely resolution or until the tests show improvement.[4] Although negativity in these tests largely excludes IgE mediated cow's milk allergy, it does not exclude non-IgE mediated cow's milk allergy.[13] The role of atopy patch testing in the diagnosis of cow's milk allergy is uncertain.[4]

Lactose intolerance, which manifests as loose watery explosive diarrhoea after ingestion of cow's milk (lactose), should be considered as part of the differential diagnosis.

Patients with severe symptoms, or in whom the diagnosis is uncertain, should be referred to a specialist (allergist, dermatologist, paediatric gastroenterologist, or general paediatrician) for further investigation and management.

How should we manage this condition?

The key to management is the elimination of cow's milk proteins from the patient's or the mother's diet (or both). Extensively hydrolysed formulas are the mainstay of such diets, although about 10% of patients are intolerant of these and require amino acid formulas.[3] [14] Other mammalian, soya, or rice milks formulas are not recommended because of high antigenic crossover. Solids must be dairy free. Dietetic advice and support are important to ensure provision of adequate nutrients to the growing child and the mother.

Symptoms may be managed with topical or systemic treatments (such as emollients and antihistamines). Patients at risk of anaphylactic reactions need adrenaline pens, along with education about their use.[15]

Challenge (usually from 12 months of age) is an important part of management, although the timing of challenge will be determined by case type and severity. Follow-up of large birth cohorts has shown that cow's milk allergy usually resolves within the first few years of life, with 60-75% of patients becoming tolerant by the age of 2 years and 84-87% by 3 years.[1] Allergy is more likely to persist in infants with IgE mediated disease and is associated with

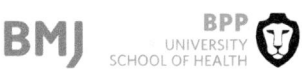

the development of other atopic conditions.[16] A normal diet can gradually be resumed after a negative challenge result.

Prevention

Strategies to prevent the development of cow's milk allergy have received considerable interest. Reviews by the American Academy of Pediatrics and the European Academy of Allergology and Clinical Immunology found evidence that exclusive breast feeding, or the use of extensively hydrolysed formulas, alongside avoidance of solids that contain dairy products, for the first four to six months reduces the incidence of the disease in infants at high risk of developing milk allergy (those with a first degree relative with physician diagnosed atopic disease).[17] [18]

Contributors: JRA wrote the article, under expert guidance and review by RMB. Both authors produced the final version. RMB is guarantor.

Competing interests: RMB has been paid as an adviser to Numico and Schering Plough and has received sponsorship from Nestle, Mead Johnson, SHS, Nutricia, and SMA to attend conferences. He has also given presentations at meetings sponsored by Nestle, SHS, and SMA.

Provenance and peer review: Commissioned; externally peer reviewed.

Patient consent not required (patient anonymised, dead, or hypothetical).

1   Host A. Frequency of cow's milk allergy in childhood. *Ann Allergy Asthma Immunol* 2002;89(6 suppl 1):33-7.
2   Macdougall CF, Cant AJ, Colver AF. How dangerous is food allergy in childhood? The incidence of severe and fatal allergic reactions across the UK and Ireland. *Arch Dis Child* 2002;86:236-9.
3   Heine R, Elsayed S, Hosking CS, Hill DJ. Cow's milk allergy in infancy. *Curr Opin Allergy Clin Immunol* 2002;2:217-25.
4   Vandenplas Y, Brueton M, Dupont C, Hill D, Isolauri E, Koletzko S, et al. Guidelines for the diagnosis and management of cow's milk protein allergy in infants. *Arch Dis Child* 2007;92:902-8.
5   Eggesbo M, Botten G, Stigum H. Restricted diets in children with reactions to milk and egg perceived by their parents. *J Pediatr* 2001;139:583-7.
6   Medeiros LC, Speridião PG, Sdepanian VL, Fagundes-Neto U, Morais MB. Nutrient intake and nutritional status of children following a diet free from cow's milk and cow's milk by-products. *J Pediatria (Rio J)* 2004;80:363-70.
7   Sampson HA, Sicherer SH, Birnbaum AH. AGA technical review on the evaluation of food allergy in gastrointestinal disorders. *Gastroenterology* 2001;120:1026-40.
8   Sicherer SH. Clinical aspects of gastrointestinal food allergy in childhood. *Pediatrics* 2003;111:1609-16.
9   National Institute for Health and Clinical Excellence. *Atopic eczema in children. Management of atopic eczema in children from birth up to age of 12 years.* 2007. www.nice.org.uk/guidance/index.jsp?action=byID&o=11636.
10 Luccassen PLBJ, Assendelft WJJ, Gubbels JW, van Eijk JTM, van Geldrop WJ, Knuistingh Neven A. Effectiveness of treatments for infantile colic: systematic review. *BMJ* 1998;316:1563-9.
11 Garrison MM, Christakis DA. A systematic review of treatments for infant colic. *Pediatrics* 2000;106:184-90.
12 Salvatore S, Vandenplas Y. Gastroesophageal reflux and cow milk allergy: is there a link? *Pediatrics* 2002;110:972-84.
13 Sicherer SH, Sampson HA. Food allergy. *J Allergy Clin Immunol* 2006;117:S470-5.
14 Høst A, Koletzko B, Dreborg S, Muraro A, Wahn U, Aggett P, et al. Dietary products used in infants for treatment and prevention of food allergy. Joint statement of the European Society for Paediatric Allergology and Clinical Immunology (ESPACI) committee on hypoallergenic formulas and the European Society for Paediatric Gastroenterology, Hepatology and Nutrition (ESPGHAN) committee on nutrition. *Arch Dis Child* 1999;81:80-4.
15 McLean-Tooke APC, Bethune CA, Fay AC, Spickett GP. Adrenaline in the treatment of anaphylaxis: what is the evidence? *BMJ* 2003;327:1332-5.
16 Høst A, Halken S, Jacobsen HP, Christensen AE, Herskind AM, Plesner K. Clinical course of cow's milk protein allergy/intolerance and atopic diseases in childhood. *Pediatr Allergy Immunol* 2002;13(suppl 15):23-8.
17 Greer FR, Sicherer SH, Burks MD, the Committee on Nutrition and Section on Allergy and Immunology. Effects of early nutritional interventions on the development of atopic disease in infants and children: the role of maternal dietary restriction, breastfeeding, timing of introduction of complementary foods, and hydrolysed formulas. *Pediatrics* 2008;121:183-91.
18 Muraro A, Dreborg S, Halken S, Høst A, Niggemann B, Aalberse R, et al. Dietary prevention of allergic diseases in infants and small children. Part III: critical review of published peer-reviewed observational and interventional studies and final recommendations. *Pediatr Allergy Immunol* 2004;15:291-307.

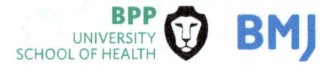

Whooping cough

Anthony Harnden, university lecturer in general practice[1]

[1]Department of Primary Health Care, University of Oxford, Oxford OX3 7LF

anthony.harnden@phc.ox.ac.uk

Cite this as: *BMJ* 2009;338:b1772

DOI: 10.1136/bmj.b1772

www.bmj.com/content/338/bmj.b1772

Whooping cough is a common respiratory infection caused by the bacterium *Bordetella pertussis*. It should be considered as a possible diagnosis in any adolescent or adult with an acute cough of more than two weeks' duration, even if they have been fully immunised.

Why is it missed?

In the post-vaccination era, whooping cough is under-recognised in primary care as the incidence is incorrectly thought to be low. The classic clinical features of whooping cough, such as an inspiratory "whoop" (listen on bmj.com), may be attenuated in older children and adults who have been immunised.[1] Moreover, many doctors may not be aware that there is a simple diagnostic serological test.

Why does this matter?

A persistent cough without explanation can cause distress and anxiety, and the patient may be subject to inappropriate investigations, treatment, and referral.[5] Secondly, early diagnosis and treatment with erythromycin can prevent the patient transmitting their infection within and outside the household.[6] This may be especially important in young infants, who may have severe complications such as respiratory failure and death.[7] Thirdly, notification of all cases of whooping cough by primary care clinicians and enhanced surveillance of laboratory proved cases would give a better estimate of the efficacy of the vaccine and of the burden of disease in the community.

How is it diagnosed?

Clinical features

Acute cough persisting for more than two weeks, without the characteristic inspiratory whoop, may be the only clinical symptom of whooping cough. Initial symptoms, lasting for up to two weeks, mimic a simple upper respiratory tract infection. This is the most infectious period. Paroxysmal episodes of coughing may continue for up to six weeks but can recur with further respiratory infections. In China whooping cough is referred to as the one hundred day cough. In all age groups, irrespective of immunisation status, the cough lasts an average of three months.

Investigations

Bordetella pertussis is a difficult organism to culture without a correctly collected pernasal swab or nasopharyngeal aspirate; neither of these samples is easy to collect in primary care. The sensitivity of culture falls from 15-45% to 0% during the first three weeks of the cough, and sensitivity may be further reduced by antibiotic treatment, previous immunisation, and transport of the specimen.[8]

KEY POINTS

- Consider a diagnosis of whooping cough in any patient with an acute persistent cough of more than two weeks' duration
- A single raised IgG titre to pertussis toxin is 99% specific for diagnosis and is the recommended test in primary care
- Oral erythromycin taken within 21 days of the onset of the cough may prevent transmission
- Notification of all cases of whooping cough by primary care clinicians, and enhanced surveillance of laboratory proved cases, would give a better estimate of vaccine efficacy and the burden of disease in the community

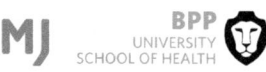

HOW COMMON IS IT?

Whooping cough is a statutory notifiable disease in the United Kingdom, but notifications remain low. Yet epidemiological evidence indicates that whooping cough remains an endemic disease in adolescents and adults.[2] International case series of adolescents and adults with cough lasting for two weeks or more have reported that about 20% of individuals have evidence of recent whooping cough.[3] Serological surveys have shown that whooping cough occurs repeatedly throughout adult life, and it has been estimated people have up to three episodes in a lifetime, despite immunisation.[4]

CASE SCENARIO

A 17 year old girl presents with a three week history of cough. The cough keeps her awake at night and she has bouts of coughing that disturb her classmates. She is fully immunised. Her general practitioner requests serology for anti-pertussis toxin IgG antibodies, which are found to be raised, indicating a recent infection with *Bordetella pertussis*.

Serology is the recommended diagnostic blood test in primary care and is routinely used in many countries: a single raised titre of antipertussis toxin IgG has a sensitivity of 76% and a specificity of 99% for the diagnosis of whooping cough across all age groups.[9] More recently, assays of antipertussis toxin IgG levels in oral fluid have been validated; they are quick and simple to use in primary care and have recently been made available in the UK.[10]

How is it managed?

Whooping cough should be notified. Treatment may not affect outcome for the patient, but erythromycin within 21 days of onset of symptoms reduces the period of infectivity and may prevent transmission to household members.[6] A seven day course is sufficient. Prophylaxis with erythromycin should be offered to everyone in households with a vulnerable infant who may be unimmunised or partly immunised.[6] In infants the illness may be severe and require prompt referral to secondary care.

I thank Doug Jenkinson for permission to use an audio clip from his website and for his work in promoting the clinical recognition of whooping cough in primary care.

Funding: No external funding.

Competing interests: AH has an ongoing interest in pertussis research and is conducting studies involving the use of oral fluid antibody testing.

Provenance and peer review: Not commissioned; externally peer reviewed.

1 Harnden A, Grant C, Harrison T, Perera R, Brueggemann AB, Mayon-White R, et al. Whooping cough in school age children with persistent cough: a prospective cohort study in primary care *BMJ* 2006;333:174-7.

2 Wright SW, Edwards KM, Decker MD, Zeldin MH. Pertussis infection in adults with persistent cough. *JAMA* 1995;273:1044-6.

3 Cagney M, MacIntyre CR, McIntyre P, Torvaldsen S, Melot V. Cough symptoms in children aged 5-14 years in Sydney, Australia: non-specific cough or unrecognized pertussis? *Respirology* 2005;10:359-64.

4 De Melker HE, Versteegh FG, Schellekens JF, Teunis PF, Kretzshmar M. The incidence of Bordetella pertussis infections estimated in the population from a combination of serological surveys. *J Infect* 2006;53:106-13.

5 Levenson R. A patient's journey: whooping cough. *BMJ* 2007;334:532-3.

6 Dodhia H, Crowcroft NS, Bramley JC, Miller E. UK guidelines for use of erythromycin chemoprophylaxis in persons exposed to pertussis. *J Public Health Med* 2002;24:200-6.

7 Crowcroft NS, Andrews N, Rooney C, Brisson M, Miller E. Deaths from pertussis are underestimated in England. *Arch Dis Child* 2002;86:336-8.

8 Crowcroft NS, Peabody RG. Recent developments in pertussis *Lancet* 2006;367:1926-36.

9 De Melker HE, Versteegh FG, Conyn-van Spaendonck, Elvers LH, berbers GA, van der Zee A, et al. Specificity and sensitivity of high levels of immunoglobulin G antibodies against pertussis toxin in a single serum sample for diagnosis of infection with Bordetella pertussis. *J Clin Microbiol* 2000;38(2):800-6.

10 Litt DJ, Samuel D, Duncan J, Harnden A, George RC, Harrison TG. Detection of anti-pertussis toxin IgG in oral fluids for use in diagnosis and surveillance of Bordetella pertussis infection in children and young adults. *J Med Microbiol* 2006;55:1223-8.

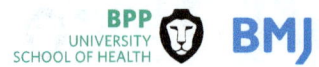

Foreign body inhalation in children

Kay Wang, senior clinical research fellow[1],
Anthony Harnden, university lecturer in general practice[1],
Anne Thomson, consultant respiratory paediatrician[2]

[1]Department of Primary Health Care, University of Oxford, Oxford OX3 7LF

[2]John Radcliffe Hospital, Oxford OX3 9DU

Correspondence to: A Thomson anne.thomson@orh.nhs.uk

Cite this as: *BMJ* 2010;341:c3924

DOI: 10.1136/bmj.c3924

www.bmj.com/content/341/bmj.c3924

Children, especially toddlers, tend to place objects in their mouths while exploring their environment. They are therefore at increased risk of inhaling foreign bodies, which may become lodged in the tracheobronchial system.

Why is it missed?

Diagnosis of an inhaled foreign body was delayed by more than a week in 29% of cases and by more than 30 days in 10% in a retrospective analysis of 1015 cases.[4] A witnessed choking event is the most important factor in pinpointing an early (within 24 hours) diagnosis of foreign body inhalation.[5] However, a consecutive series of 142 children attending a hospital emergency department with a history suggesting foreign body inhalation found that such events are not reported in 1 in 6 (10/61) confirmed cases.[6] Parents or carers may not witness or remember choking episodes, and children may not disclose a history of choking or of inhaling foreign bodies because of limited speech, fear or embarrassment.

Clinicians may fail to consider the diagnosis of an inhaled foreign body if the child has no symptoms at presentation or presents with prolonged or atypical symptoms, especially when physical examination and chest radiograph findings are normal.[7] Inhaled objects that do not cause an intense inflammatory response (plastic toys, for example) or that result in only partial airway occlusion are the most difficult to detect.

Why does it matter?

Delayed diagnosis of an inhaled foreign body can result in complete airway obstruction, which may be fatal.[3] The rate of serious acute complications (including pneumonia, pneumothorax, and subglottic oedema) is 2.5 times higher when diagnosed more than 24 hours after inhalation (67%) than when diagnosed within 24 hours (27%).[8] Long term complication rates are also higher if diagnosis is delayed. In one follow-up study (almost 30% (6/21)) of children in whom foreign body removal was delayed by more than one week developed a chronic persistent cough (mean duration of follow-up 2.05 years).[9] Recurrent pneumonia, lung abscesses, and bronchiectasis can also develop if foreign bodies remain in place for many weeks.[10]

How is it diagnosed?

Clinical features

The table lists the sensitivities, specificities, and positive and negative predictive values of clinical features associated with foreign body inhalation in children. In a 10 year chart review, 77 out of 135 children (57%) showed the classic triad of coughing or choking,

---

KEY POINTS

- A diagnosis of foreign body inhalation should be considered in any child in whom a witnessed choking episode is reported
- Clinicians should specifically ask about previous choking episodes in children presenting with persistent cough or other respiratory symptoms
- Bronchoscopy is recommended in children with a suggestive history together with symptoms, signs, or chest radiograph findings consistent with foreign body inhalation; an index of suspicion should be maintained in children with a suggestive history only

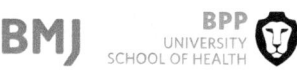

Table 1 Diagnostic value of clinical findings in foreign body inhalation

Findings	Sensitivity (%)	Specificity (%)	Positive predictive value (%)	Negative predictive value (%)
History of witnessed choking event[6]	92	32	50	84
Cough[6]	92	28	49	82
Wheeze[12]	88	28	76	47
Dyspnoea[12]	18	74	64	26
Localised decreased lung sounds[6]	57	85	74	73

CASE SCENARIO

A 2 year old boy presented to his general practitioner with a two week history of a dry, persistent cough. His mother recalled an episode two weeks ago when he had a violent coughing fit while eating nuts and raisins. She took him to the nearest hospital emergency department, but he was discharged a few hours later after a normal physical examination and normal chest radiograph. Nevertheless, this history of persistent cough following a choking episode should raise concern about possible foreign body inhalation.

HOW COMMON IS IT?

- During 2008-9, just over 300 hospital admissions in England were due to foreign body inhalation in children up to 14 years of age[1]

- Worldwide, 55% of children who have inhaled foreign bodies are between 1 and 3 years of age and 7-10% are under 1 year of age[2]

- In the United States, foreign body inhalation accounts for 7% of accidental deaths in children under 4 years of age[3]

---

wheezing, and unilateral reduced breath sounds.[7] Wheeze is present when there is partial obstruction of an airway. Persistent cough, wheeze, sputum production, and dyspnoea may develop in children in whom diagnosis is delayed by more than one month.[11]

Investigations

Chest radiograph findings compatible with an inhaled foreign body include air trapping, atelectasis, and pneumothorax. After several days, radiographic evidence of pneumonia may also be present. However, none of these findings are pathognomonic for foreign body inhalation.[13] In addition, more than three quarters of inhaled foreign bodies are radiolucent and will therefore not show on chest radiographs.[14]

Definitive diagnosis of foreign body inhalation is by endoscopic evaluation. The most appropriate first line procedure depends on the likelihood of a foreign body being present. Where there is near certainty, rigid bronchoscopy under general anaesthesia is the investigation of choice, as the object can be detected and removed in one procedure.[6] In cases where clinical and radiographic findings are equivocal, flexible bronchoscopy under sedation and local anaesthesia can be useful in confirming the presence and exact site of the item.[2] Subsequent removal is by rigid bronchoscopy under general anaesthesia.

How is it managed?

Bronchoscopy is recommended when children have a suggestive history together with symptoms, signs, or chest radiograph findings consistent with foreign body inhalation. Children with a suggestive history but normal clinical and chest radiograph findings should be monitored carefully for symptoms and signs of foreign body inhalation.[6] Given the considerable mortality and morbidity associated with foreign body inhalation in children, the importance of preventive measures needs to be emphasised to parents and carers.

Contributors: KW wrote the first draft of the article, which was modified by AH and AT. All authors agreed on the final draft. AT is guarantor.

Funding: KW's post is funded by the National Institute for Health Research.

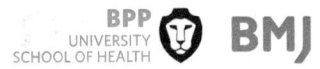

Competing interests: AT has given a presentation for Kayonesse Conferences on cough and wheeze in children for which financial payment was received by AT's academic institution.

Provenance and peer review: Not commissioned; externally peer reviewed.

1   Hospital Episode Statistics. External cause, 2008-9. http://www.hesonline.nhs.uk/Ease/servlet/ContentServer?siteID=1937&categoryID=211.

2   Righini CA, Morel N, Karkas A, Reyt E, Ferretti K, Pin I, et al. What is the diagnostic value of flexible bronchoscopy in the initial investigation of children with suspected foreign body aspiration? *Int J Pediatr Otorhinolaryngol* 2007;71:1383-90.

3   Mantor PC, Tuggle DW, Tunell WP. An appropriate negative bronchoscopy rate in suspected foreign body aspiration. *Am J Surg* 1989;158:622-4.

4   Saki N, Nikakhlagh S, Rahim F, Abshirini H. Foreign body aspirations in infancy: a 20-year experience. *Int J Med Sci* 2009;6:322-8.

5   Chiu C-Y, Wong K-S, Lai S-H, Hsia S-H, Wu C-T. Factors predicting early diagnosis of foreign body aspiration in children. *Pediatr Emerg Care* 2005;21:161-4.

6   Cohen S, Avital A, Godfrey S, Gross M, Kerem E, Springer C. Suspected foreign body inhalation in children: what are the indications for bronchoscopy? *J Pediatr* 2009;155:276-80.

7   Tan HKK, Brown K, McGill T, Kenna MA, Lund DP, Healy GB. Airway foreign bodies (FB): a 10-year review. *Int J Pediatr Otorhinolaryngol* 2000;56:91-9.

8   Esclamado RM, Richardson MA. Laryngotracheal foreign bodies in children: a comparison with bronchial foreign bodies. *Am J Dis Child* 1987;141:259-62.

9   Davies H, Gordon I, Matthew DJ, Helms P, Kenney IJ, Lutkin JE, et al. Long term follow up after inhalation of foreign bodies. *Arch Dis Child* 1990;65:619-21.

10 Abdulmajid OA, Ebeid AM, Motaweh MM, Kleibo IS. Aspirated foreign bodies in the tracheobronchial tree: report of 250 cases. *Thorax* 1976;31:635-40.

11 Karakoc F, Cakir E, Ersu R, Uyan ZS, Colak B, Karadag B, et al. Late diagnosis of foreign body aspiration in children with chronic respiratory symptoms. *Int J Pediatr Otorhinolaryngol* 2007;71:241-6.

12 Kiyan G, Gocmen B, Tugtepe H, Karakoc F, Dagli E, Dagli TE. Foreign body aspiration in children: The value of diagnostic criteria. *Int J Pediatr Otorhinolaryngol* 2009;73:963-7.

13 Svedstrom E, Puhakka H, Kero P. How accurate is chest radiography in the diagnosis of tracheobronchial foreign bodies in children? *Pediatr Radiol* 1989;19:520-2.

14 Sersar SI, Rizk WH, Bilal M, El Diasty MM, Eltantawy TA, Abdelhakam BB, et al. Inhaled foreign bodies: presentation, management and value of history and plain chest radiography in delayed presentation. *Otolaryngol Head Neck Surg* 2006;134:92-7.

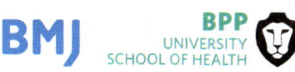

Kawasaki disease

Anthony Harnden, professor of primary care[1],
Robert Tulloh, professor of congenital cardiology[2],
David Burgner, professor[3]

[1]Department of Primary Care Health Sciences, University of Oxford, Oxford, UK

[2]University Hospitals Bristol NHS Foundation Trust, University of Bristol, Bristol, UK

[3]Murdoch Childrens Research Institute and Department of Paediatrics, University of Melbourne, Parkville, VIC, Australia

Correspondence to: anthony.harnden@phc.ox.ac.uk

Cite this as: BMJ 2014;349:g5336

DOI: 10.1136/bmj.g5336

www.bmj.com/content/338/bmj.b1514

Case scenario

A 2 year old boy was brought to see the general practitioner by his parents because of a four day history of fever. His parents noticed a rash and slightly "bloodshot" eyes the day before. The GP diagnosed a viral illness, offered reassurance, but gave good safety netting advice. The boy re-presented to his GP three days later, still intermittently febrile, irritable, and with an angry looking widespread morbilliform rash and a sore mouth. Kawasaki disease was suspected, and he was admitted to hospital where he received prompt treatment with intravenous immunoglobulin and high dose aspirin. An echocardiogram, performed during admission was normal, as were those during follow-up.

What is Kawasaki disease?

Kawasaki disease is an acute inflammatory vasculitis of medium size arteries that occurs mainly in children aged 6 months to 5 years but can occur at any age, including younger infants, and even occasionally in adults.[1][2][3] Although one or multiple infectious triggers are most likely, the precise cause is unclear. Kawasaki disease is the commonest cause of acquired heart disease in children in industrialised countries because the coronary arteries are affected in about a quarter of untreated cases. The incidence of acquired heart disease in children is rising.[4]

Why is Kawasaki disease missed?

A recent observational study of Kawasaki disease set in primary care reported a delay of more than 10 days (range of the time for the total sample between GP presentation and admission was 0-86 days) between first presentation and hospital admission for 7% of children.[11] In the initial stages the fever and rash of Kawasaki disease can mimic viral exanthemata, such as parvovirus, adenovirus, and measles, as well as group A streptococcal infection. Parents might be falsely reassured that their child has a simple febrile illness and delay seeking further advice when symptoms persist or new symptoms appear. In any infant under 6 months, a prolonged fever of seven days or more, with laboratory evidence of inflammation, should be considered as Kawasaki disease and be referred for assessment and possible treatment.[12]

KEY POINTS

- Consider a diagnosis of Kawasaki disease in young children with irritability and prolonged fever (>5 days) and refer to hospital for assessment and treatment
- Incomplete Kawasaki disease—fever but fewer than four of the other diagnostic criteria (bilateral conjuntival injection, polymorphous exanthema, changes to the extremities or lips and oral cavity or both)—represents 15-20% of cases
- Treatment with intravenous immunoglobulin within five to 10 days of fever onset reduces the incidence of coronary artery lesions from 25% to ~5%
- A transthoracic echocardiogram is essential to identify coronary artery abnormalities, assess myocardial and valvular function, and exclude clinically important pericardial effusion, but a normal study does not exclude Kawasaki disease

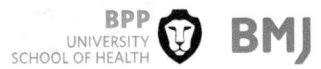
> ### THE DIAGNOSTIC FEATURES OF KAWASAKI DISEASE[12]
>
> Fever (>39°C) for at least four days and at least four of the following features, after exclusion of other similar diseases*
>
> - Bilateral non-exudative bulbar conjunctival injection
> - Polymorphous exanthema
> - Changes in the extremities (acute—erythema of palms and soles, oedema of hands and feet. Subacute—periungual peeling of fingers and toes)
> - Changes to lips and oral cavity (red, fissured lips, strawberry tongue, erythema of oropharyngeal mucosa, without exudates)
> - Cervical lymphadenopathy (≥1.5 cm, usually unilateral, rare in infants)

> ### HOW COMMON IS KAWASAKI DISEASE?
>
> - England—8.39 per 100 000 children under 5 years[5]
> - Australia—9.34 per 100 000 children under 5 years[6]
> - Japan—239 per 100 000 children under 5 years[7]
> - Korea—134 per 100 000 children under 5 years[8]
> - Taiwan—66 per 100 000 children under 5 years[9]
> - Hawaii—210 per 100 000 Japanese American children under 5 years, and 13 per 100 000 white children under 5 years[10]

Why does it matter?

Kawasaki disease can cause damage and dilation of the coronary arteries, including aneurysms. These may be small, but in some, there can be substantial dilation or even giant aneurysms (>8 mm internal diameter). These can thrombose acutely or can heal with stenosis, causing myocardial ischaemia many months or years later.[13] In addition, there might be acute myocarditis, leading to poor heart function, valvular regurgitation, or pericardial effusion.

It is important that Kawasaki disease is diagnosed early because treatment with intravenous immunoglobulin within five to 10 days of fever onset reduces the incidence of coronary artery lesions from 25% to ~5%.[12] [13] Delays in treatment might lead to unnecessary morbidity and occasionally death. The mortality rate is about 0.2% and is most commonly secondary to thrombosis of giant aneurysms or later myocardial ischaemia and infarction.[12] Infants under 6 months, who have had fever for seven days or more, are often diagnosed late owing to incomplete features, and they might have serious, potentially life-threatening complications.[14]

How is Kawasaki disease diagnosed?

Clinical features

The diagnosis of Kawasaki disease is made on clinical grounds. Fever is universal and typically unresponsive to antipyretics and antibiotics. The diagnostic clinical criteria are individually insensitive and non-specific. Definite Kawasaki disease is characterised by prolonged fever (usually defined as ≥5 days) and at least four out of five key diagnostic features (box). Children with prolonged fever and suspected Kawasaki disease should be referred promptly for further assessment.

The clinical features often occur sequentially and some might have resolved by presentation, so a focused history is essential. Children who have been vaccinated with BCG might have inflammation at the vaccination site. Children with Kawasaki disease are often noticeably irritable. Incomplete Kawasaki disease (fever but less than four diagnostic criteria) is common (15-20% of all cases), so a high index of suspicion is needed for any young child or infant with prolonged fever and no clear diagnosis. Incomplete Kawasaki

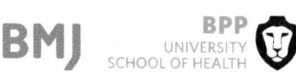

disease is associated with increased incidence of coronary artery abnormalities, possibly caused by delayed diagnosis.[12 14]

Investigations

No diagnostic test is available for Kawasaki disease. Laboratory features can aid the diagnosis but, as with the clinical diagnostic criteria, they lack individual specificity and sensitivity. Leucocytosis and neutrophilia are usually found. Thrombocytosis is common but occurs subacutely (week two to three), so it is not helpful diagnostically. Inflammatory markers are typically raised and mild abnormalities of liver function tests are common. White blood cells are often present in the (sterile) urine or cerebrospinal fluid, or both. A microbiologically confirmed infection is also present in a third of patients with Kawasaki disease and should not preclude the diagnosis.[15]

A transthoracic echocardiogram is essential to identify coronary artery abnormalities, assess myocardial and valvular function, and exclude a clinically important pericardial effusion. These changes might be identified at presentation in severe cases but usually develop in the subacute phase (2-3 weeks). Echocardiography is therefore not useful diagnostically, and a normal study should not influence the decision to treat Kawasaki disease. Echocardiography is performed at presentation, with follow-up echocardiograms at two weeks—if there is concern—six weeks, and often at six months. Subjective brightness of the walls of the coronary arteries, mild dilation (ectasia), or frank aneurysms might be seen.[16]

How is Kawasaki disease managed?

Hospital admission is necessary. On the basis of randomised control trials, intravenous polyclonal immunoglobulin has become the established treatment, and it reduces the risk of coronary artery aneurysms from 25% to less than 5%.[12 17] Aspirin is given, although dosing regimens vary.[17 18] Additional corticosteroids have been recommended in some countries for severe and evolving cases.[17] About 15% of patients do not respond to immunoglobulin, and subsequent treatment often comprises a second infusion of immunoglobulin and intravenous methylprednisolone.[12 17 19]

Most children in industrialised countries have few long term sequelae if treated promptly and appropriately. A small proportion of children with major coronary artery damage will require ongoing specialist management. Some patients report behavioural changes and desquamation of fingers and toes with subsequent febrile illness.[20] Live vaccines (such as measles, mumps, and rubella) should be delayed for 11 months after treatment with intravenous immunoglobulin. Recurrence is rare (<1%), the risk in siblings is probably modestly increased (about 10 times the population risk in Japan).[12] Kawasaki disease is not contagious. Families of children with this disease might benefit from follow-up with a doctor familiar with the condition to allay anxiety and answer specific queries, even if there are no long term coronary artery abnormalities.

Competing interests: We have read and understood the BMJ policy on declaration of interests and declare the following interests: DB has salary and support for research into Kawasaki disease from the National Health and Medical Research Council, and Murdoch Childrens Research Institute; he also has invitations (partly reimbursed) to present Kawasaki disease-related research findings at conferences of the European Society for Paediatric Infectious Diseases, World Society for Paediatric Infectious Diseases, International Kawasaki Disease Symposia, and the World Congress of Cardiology; DB is also involved in the preparation of educational material for the Kawasaki Disease Foundation, Australia. None of these agencies or bodies had any input or influence over the manuscript at any stage. AH and RT have no interests to declare.

Provenance and peer review: not commissioned; externally peer reviewed.

Patient consent not required (patient anonymised, dead, or hypothetical).

1   Burns JC, Glodé MP. Kawasaki syndrome. *Lancet* 2004;364:533-44.
2   Harnden A, Takahashi M, Burgner D. Kawasaki disease. *BMJ* 2009;338:b1514.

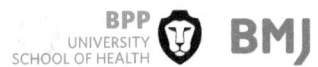

3   Yim D, Curtis N, Cheung M, Burgner D. An update on Kawasaki disease II: clinical features, diagnosis, treatment and outcomes. *J Paediatr Child Health* 2013;49:614-23.

4   Yim D, Curtis N, Cheung M, Burgner D Update on Kawasaki disease: epidemiology, aetiology and pathogenesis. *J Paediatr Child Health* 2013;49:704-8.

5   Harnden A, Mayon-White R, Perera R, Yeates D, Goldacre M, Burgner D. Kawasaki disease in England: ethnicity, deprivation, and respiratory pathogens. *Pediatr Infect Dis J* 2009;28:21-4.

6   Saundankar J, Yim D, Itotoh B, Payne R, Maslin K, Jape G, et al. The epidemiology and clinical features of Kawasaki disease in Australia. *Pediatrics* 2014;133:e1009-14.

7   Nakamura Y, Yashiro M, Uehara R, Sadakane A, Tsuboi S, Aoyama, et al. Epidemiologic features of Kawasaki disease in Japan: results of the 2009-2010 nationwide survey. *J Epidemiol* 2012;22:216-21.

8   Kim GB, Han JW, Park YW, Song MS, Hong YM, Cha SH, et al. Epidemiologic features of Kawasaki disease in South Korea: data from nationwide survey, 2009-2011. *Pediatr Infect Dis J* 2014;33:24-7.

9   Lue HC, Chen LR, Lin MT, Chang LY, Wang JK, Lee CY, et al. Epidemiological features of Kawasaki disease in Taiwan, 1976-2007: results of five nationwide questionnaire hospital surveys. *Pediatr Neonatol* 2014;55:92-6.

10 Holman RC, Christensen KY, Belay ED, Steiner CA, Effler PV, Miyamura J, et al. Racial/ethnic differences in the incidence of Kawasaki syndrome among children in Hawaii. *Hawaii Med J* 2010;69:194-7.

11 Moore A, Harnden A, Mayon-White R. Recognising Kawasaki Disease in UK primary care: a descriptive study using the Clinical Practice Research Datalink. *Br J Gen Pract* 2014;64:e477-83.

12 Newburger JW, Takahashi M, Gerber MA, Gewitz MH, Tani LY, Burns JC, et al Diagnosis, treatment, and long-term management of Kawasaki disease: a statement for health professionals from the Committee on Rheumatic Fever, Endocarditis, and Kawasaki Disease, Council on Cardiovascular Disease in the Young, American Heart Association. *Pediatrics* 2004:114:1708-33.

13 Tsuda E, Hamaoka K, Suzuki H, Sakazaki H, Murakami Y, Nakagawa M, et al. A survey of the 3-decade outcome for patients with giant aneurysms caused by Kawasaki disease. *Am Heart J* 2014;167:249-58.

14 Yeom JS, Woo HO, Park JS, Park ES, Seo JH, Youn HS. Kawasaki disease in infants. *Korean J Pediatr* 2013;56:377-82.

15 Benseler SM, McCrindle BW, Silverman ED, Tyrrell PN, Wong J, Yeung RS. Infections and Kawasaki disease: implications for coronary artery outcome. *Pediatrics* 2005;116:e760-6.

16 Wood LE, Tulloh RM. Kawasaki disease in children. *Heart* 2009;95:787-92.

17 Eleftheriou D, Levin M, Shingadia D, Tulloh R, Klein N, Brogan P. Management of Kawasaki disease. *Arch Dis Child* 2014;99:74-83.

18 Yim D, Curtis N, Cheung M, Burgner D.An update on Kawasaki disease II: clinical features, diagnosis, treatment and outcomes. *J Paediatr Child Health* 2013;49:614-23.

19 Tacke CE, Burgner D, Kuipers IM, Kuijpers TW. Management of acute and refractory Kawasaki disease. *Expert Rev Anti Infect Ther* 2012;10:1203-15.

20 Tacke CE, Haverman L, Berk BM, van Rossum MA, Kuipers IM, Grootenhuis MA, et al. Quality of life and behavioral functioning in Dutch children with a history of Kawasaki disease. *J Pediatr* 2012;161:314-9.

Related links

thebmj.com/archive

Previous articles in this series
- Postnatal depression (BMJ 2014;349:g4500)
- Motor neurone disease (BMJ 2014;349:g4052)
- Copper deficiency (BMJ 2014;348:g3691)
- Bladder cancer in women (BMJ 2014;348:g2171)
- Subdural haematoma in the elderly (BMJ 2014;348:g1682)

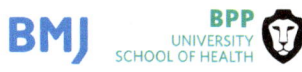

Septic arthritis in children

Andrew Howard, consultant paediatric orthopaedic surgeon[1],
Mary Wilson, family practitioner[2]

[1]Division of Orthopaedic Surgery, Hospital for Sick Children, 555 University Avenue, Toronto, ON, Canada M5G1X8

[2]Marathon Family Health Team, Marathon, ON, Canada

Correspondence to: A Howard andrew.howard@sickkids.ca

Cite this as: BMJ 2010;341:c4407

DOI: 10.1136/bmj.c4407

www.bmj.com/content/341/bmj.c4407

A differential diagnosis of septic arthritis in children can be difficult, but early treatment of joint infections avoids potentially disabling complications.

Septic arthritis accounts for a small minority of the myriad musculoskeletal problems in childhood which primary care doctors will evaluate. Joint infections are best treated early to avoid potentially disabling complications. The earlier the presentation, the more difficult it is to distinguish an infection from benign, self limited conditions such as transient synovitis of the hip.

Why is it missed?

Joint infections overlap in presentation with transient synovitis, unexplained symptoms, and minor trauma, all of which are common. Musculoskeletal infections in very young children and in very ill children can be missed because the symptoms and signs that localise the problem are absent. Untreated pyogenic infection eventually "declares itself," but this may be too late for optimal treatment. Antibiotic treatment before diagnosis (prescribed for other conditions or empirically) may mask clinical findings without curing the disease.

Why does this matter?

Missed septic arthritis results in severe destruction of the child's hip, which is difficult to treat.[3] [4] A prospective cohort study of all children presenting with septic arthritis of the hip in South Africa found no sequelae among children diagnosed and treated within five days of onset of symptoms, but a very high incidence of permanent problems among those treated at five days or later.[5] Late treatment cannot reverse the damage, caused by pus under pressure and compromised blood flow, to the joint cartilage, the epiphyseal bone, or the growth plate. Unfortunately, more than two thirds of the children in the South African series were treated late, with delay in diagnosis (rather than delay in presentation) the most common reason for delay in treatment. Diagnostic delay may be less common in high income countries, but our paediatric orthopaedic unit treats many patients with ongoing sequelae of septic arthritis and sees 5-10 new late cases every year.

How is it diagnosed?

The presentation of septic arthritis is fever with limb pain, limp, or refusal to bear weight. The affected joint is held in the position of comfort, which maximises intracapsular volume. At the hip, flexion, abduction, and external rotation are typical. Muscle spasm or pain with attempts to internally rotate or "log roll" the affected hip indicates effusion, but does not distinguish septic arthritis from transient synovitis.

KEY POINTS

- Septic arthritis in children can be difficult to diagnose, and to distinguish from more common conditions such as minor trauma or transient synovitis of the hip
- Early diagnosis and treatment of septic arthritis is important to avoid joint destruction and disability
- Fever, weightbearing status, white cell count, erythrocyte sedimentation rate, and C reactive protein are considered together for diagnosis
- Children with two or more "positive" diagnostic criteria should be referred for prompt evaluation by a specialist, whereas children with no or one positive criterion can safely be watched

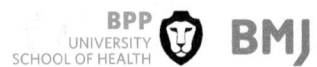

CASE SCENARIO

A 5 year old boy is brought to the accident and emergency department with pain in his left leg. The previous day he limped markedly and now he refuses to walk. History is negative for injury and positive for fever in a previously well, immunised child who is developmentally normal. Concerned about septic arthritis, the junior doctor requests a blood count, erythrocyte sedimentation rate, and C reactive protein concentration, and requests review by the paediatric team.

HOW COMMON IS IT?

- Transient synovitis is a common idiopathic inflammatory condition of the child's hip which presents in a similar manner to the "do not miss" diagnosis of septic arthritis
- Transient synovitis was diagnosed in 43 Norwegian children per 100 000 annually, compared with only five cases of septic arthritis per 100 000[1]
- Septic arthritis in children affects the hip in a third of cases, the knee in a third, and other joints in the remaining third[2]
- Septic arthritis can occur at any age in childhood but is most common among infants, toddlers, and children of preschool age[2]

The younger the child, the more difficult the clinical examination. Neonates may have few localised signs and a blunted systemic response, presenting instead with "pseudoparalysis" of the affected limb.

No single test can reliably distinguish infection from inflammation, and this has led to diagnostic algorithms combining criteria. Kocher proposed the first such algorithm, identifying refusal to bear weight, fever >38.5°C, erythrocyte sedimentation rate >40 mm/h, and white blood cell count >12.0×10⁹/l as four criteria distinguishing septic arthritis from transient synovitis.[6] If none of these criteria was positive, the probability of septic arthritis was less than 0.2%; probability rose to 3% if one criterion was positive, 40% if two were, 96% if three were, and 99% if four were. Subsequent prospective studies showed reduced but still acceptable diagnostic performance (area under receiver operating curve 0.86)[7]; other researchers have added C reactive protein >200 mg/l or a history of a previous healthcare visit to improve diagnostic accuracy.[8] [9]

Plain radiography shows nothing for the vast majority of children presenting with transient synovitis or septic arthritis. In general practice, plain radiographs are not a first line test, except in children 9 years and over to look for slipped upper femoral epiphysis.[10]

Ultrasound scans are sensitive to hip joint effusion but cannot distinguish septic arthritis from transient synovitis. They give many false negative results in early presentations or in bilateral disease.[11]

Blood cultures can be obtained but are positive only about 30% of the time.[2] Usually the child is being treated before any culture results come back.

A practical approach in primary care is to consider a complete blood count, erythrocyte sedimentation rate, and C reactive protein in any child who refuses to walk or who has a high fever with bone or joint pain or tenderness. The indications for drawing blood have not been studied, but the paper by Kocher (based on data from tertiary care) showed that of 82 children with septic arthritis, 78 refused to walk and four could walk with a limp, whereas of 86 with transient synovitis only 30 refused to walk.[6] In Kocher's series the mean recorded temperature for patients with septic arthritis was 38.7°C, compared with 37.4°C among patients with transient synovitis.

When blood is drawn, white cell count, erythrocyte sedimentation rate, C reactive protein, non-weightbearing, and fever constitute separate diagnostic criteria. If none or one diagnostic criterion (red flags) is positive, the child can be safely sent home and reviewed in 24 to 48 hours provided that parents can bring the child for re-evaluation if the condition

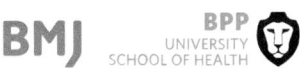

worsens. We typically advise parents to give ibuprofen and restrict activity for such children. If two or more diagnostic criteria are present, or if the child's condition worsens, a specialist should be consulted. The diagnosis is confirmed by finding pus on aspiration of the joint.

How is it managed?

Septic arthritis is managed in consultation with an orthopaedic surgeon. Management includes arthrotomy to decompress the joint, remove infected material, and reduce the chances of sequelae from avascular necrosis or damage to the growth plate. Ideally arthrotomy is performed promptly and antibiotics are begun only after intraoperative cultures are taken (or before this on the advice of the surgeon). Although recent case series have shown acceptable results with repeated joint aspiration alone,[12] [13] there is insufficient evidence to recommend this as routine practice. The current practice of the orthopaedic author (AH) includes arthrotomy in all cases of hip joint sepsis, and in most cases of sepsis of the knee or shoulder.

Contributors: AH and MW collaborated on the research, deriving clinical recommendations, and writing. AH is guarantor.

Competing interests: All authors have completed the unified competing interest form at www.icmje. org/coi_disclosure.pdf (available on request from the corresponding author) and declare no support from any organisation for the submitted work; no financial relationships with any organisation that might have an interest in the submitted work in the previous three years; and no other relationships or activities that could appear to have influenced the submitted work.

Provenance and peer review: Not commissioned; externally peer reviewed.

Patient consent not required (patient anonymised, dead, or hypothetical).

1   Riise OR, Handeland KS, Cvancarova M, Wathne KO, Nakstad B, Abrahamsen TG, et al. Incidence and characteristics of arthritis in Norwegian children: a population-based study. *Pediatrics* 2008;121:e299-306.
2   Goergens ED, McEvoy A, Watson M, Barrett IR. Acute osteomyelitis and septic arthritis in children. *J Paediatr Child Health* 2005;41:59-62.
3   Choi IH, Shin YW, Chung CY, Cho TJ, Yoo WJ, Lee DY. Surgical treatment of the severe sequelae of infantile septic arthritis of the hip. *Clin Orthop RelatRes* 2005 (434):102-9.
4   Forlin E, Milani C. Sequelae of septic arthritis of the hip in children: a new classification and a review of 41 hips. *J Pediatr Orthop* 2008;28:524-8.
5   Nunn TR, Cheung WY, Rollinson PD. A prospective study of pyogenic sepsis of the hip in childhood. *J Bone Joint Surg [Br]* 2007;89:100-6.
6   Kocher MS, Zurakowski D, Kasser JR. Differentiating between septic arthritis and transient synovitis of the hip in children: an evidence-based clinical prediction algorithm. *J Bone Joint Surg [Am]* 1999;81:1662-70.
7   Kocher MS, Mandiga R, Zurakowski D, Barnewolt C, Kasser JR. Validation of a clinical prediction rule for the differentiation between septic arthritis and transient synovitis of the hip in children. *J Bone Joint Surg [Am]* 2004;86:1629-35.
8   Caird MS, Flynn JM, Leung YL, Millman JE, D'Italia JG, Dormans JP. Factors distinguishing septic arthritis from transient synovitis of the hip in children. A prospective study. *J Bone Joint Surg [Am]* 2006;88:1251-7.
9   Luhmann SJ, Jones A, Schootman M, Gordon JE, Schoenecker PL, Luhmann JD. Differentiation between septic arthritis and transient synovitis of the hip in children with clinical prediction algorithms. *J Bone Joint Surg [Am]* 2004;86:956-62.
10 Baskett A, Hosking J, Aickin R. Hip radiography for the investigation of nontraumatic, short duration hip pain presenting to a children's emergency department. *Pediatr Emerg Care* 2009;25:78-82.
11 Gordon JE, Huang M, Dobbs M, Luhmann SJ, Szymanski DA, Schoenecker PL. Causes of false-negative ultrasound scans in the diagnosis of septic arthritis of the hip in children. *J Pediatr Orthop* 2002;22:312-6.
12 Givon U, Liberman B, Schindler A, Blankstein A, Ganel A. Treatment of septic arthritis of the hip joint by repeated ultrasound-guided aspirations. *J Pediatr Orthop* 2004;24:266-70.
13 Peltola H, Paakkonen M, Kallio P, Kallio MJ. Osteomyelitis-Septic Arthritis [OM-SA] Study Group. Prospective, randomized trial of 10 days versus 30 days of antimicrobial treatment, including a short-term course of parenteral therapy, for childhood septic arthritis. *Clin Infect Dis* 2009;48:1201-10.

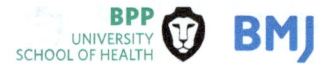

Type 1 diabetes in children

Keya Ali, consultant paediatrician[1],
Anthony Harnden, university lecturer in general practice and general practitioner[2], Julie A Edge, consultant in paediatric diabetes[1]

Type 1 diabetes in childhood is one of the commoner long term conditions of childhood. It is treated by specialist teams in secondary care using increasingly intensive insulin regimens, but the onset is generally diagnosed by primary care physicians, sometimes later than is ideal.

[1]Oxford Children's Hospital, John Radcliffe Hospital, Oxford OX3 9DU

[2]Department of Primary Health Care, Oxford OX3 7LF

Correspondence to:
J A Edge julie.edge@ paediatrics.ox.ac.uk

Cite this as: *BMJ* 2011;342:d294

DOI: 10.1136/bmj.d294

www.bmj.com/ content/342/bmj.d294

Why is it missed?

About 30% of children with newly diagnosed diabetes have had at least one related medical visit before the diagnosis, suggesting that medical practitioners are missing the diagnosis.[5] Drinking a lot and passing a lot of urine may not be mentioned by parents, even when children start bed wetting after having been dry. Other early symptoms of diabetes in young children (headache, constipation, oral and vulval thrush, abdominal pain, vomiting) may be non-specific. In older children and adolescents, polyuria and polydipsia usually predominate, but these symptoms can be misinterpreted by parents and schools or ignored by adolescents. Doctors may not consider the diagnosis as a cause of the initial symptoms; they may fail to ask about polyuria and polydipsia in children with other suggestive symptoms or may fail to carry out the appropriate investigation. Incorrect diagnoses in children with newly presenting diabetes include respiratory infection, simple candidiasis, gastroenteritis, urinary tract infection, stomatitis, and appendicitis.[6]

Why does this matter?

Children can develop dehydration and acidosis within 24 hours of first presentation, and children aged under 2 years are most at risk. In a recent UK study, a higher proportion of children with delayed diagnosis presented in diabetic ketoacidosis than did those with no delay (52% v 21%).[7] Diabetic ketoacidosis is the leading cause of mortality and morbidity in children with type 1 diabetes mellitus; 10 children a year die from diabetic ketoacidosis in the UK. Most diabetes related deaths are due to cerebral oedema, which is more common when diabetic ketoacidosis occurs at onset of diabetes.[8]

How is type 1 diabetes diagnosed in children?

Clinical features

Clinical features can be non-specific in children under 2 years, and a high index of suspicion is important. Polyuria and polydipsia are the main symptoms of diabetes in all age groups, occurring in up to three quarters of school age children.[9] However, these symptoms are

---

KEY POINTS

- Secondary nocturnal enuresis is the commonest symptom of new diabetes in children
- Ask about polyuria and polydipsia in toddlers with constipation, thrush, vomiting, weight loss, or any acute illness
- Investigate children with polyuria, polydipsia, and weight loss for diabetes
- Investigation for diabetes requires only a single immediate capillary blood glucose test; values above 11.1 mmol/L indicate diabetes
- Refer children with a raised blood glucose concentration to secondary care the same day
- Do not wait for a fasting blood glucose test or urine sample as this may allow diabetic ketoacidosis to intervene

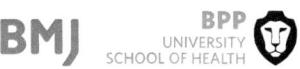

CASE SCENARIO

A 7 year old boy with acute abdominal pain and vomiting is brought to see his general practitioner by his mother. He was being bullied at school, and because his mother attributed his recent onset of bed wetting to stress she did not mention this symptom to the GP. The GP considers appendicitis a possibility but first decides to rule out a urinary tract infection. A urine dipstick test is positive for glucose and ketones. She refers the child at once to the paediatric team for immediate management of his diabetic ketoacidosis.

HOW COMMON IS IT?

- In England diabetes occurs in 1 in 450 children, of whom 97% have type 1 diabetes mellitus[1]

- The current incidence is around 26/100000 per year

- In a large UK general practice, a child with new diabetes will be seen about every two years

- Incidence is increasing by around 4% a year in the UK, in common with other northern European countries[2]

- The prevalence of diabetic ketoacidosis at diagnosis over the past 20 years has remained unchanged, at around 25% of newly diagnosed children of all ages and 35% in children under 5 years[3][4]

---

not always mentioned initially and must be elicited by a proper history taking. Nocturnal enuresis in a previously "dry" child is the earliest symptom of diabetes in 89% of children over the age of 4 years.[9][10] Weight loss occurs in half those aged 10-14 years but in only 5% of children under 2 years. Lethargy occurs in 10-20% of children of all ages. Constipation is an important symptom in the under 5s, occurring in around 10%, secondary to chronic dehydration.[9] Recurrent infections are uncommon as a presentation, occurring in only 2%, although oral and vulval thrush has been reported. Positive predictive values of these symptoms are not known as the appropriate research has not been carried out.

If ketoacidosis has already supervened, then the symptoms can include vomiting, deep sighing respiration, reduced conscious level, and abdominal pain. Because of these, diabetic ketoacidosis can be misdiagnosed as acute abdomen, possible gastroenteritis, acute asthma, or pneumonia if the parents are not asked about a history of polyuria and polydipsia.

Investigations

Diabetes can be diagnosed with a single capillary blood glucose test if a proper technique has been followed—that is, the child's hands have been washed and dried thoroughly. The diagnostic criteria for diabetes are the same in children as in adults: a random blood glucose concentration >11.1 mmol/L. Any delay obtaining a urine sample or a glucose measurement may allow diabetic ketoacidosis to supervene. If symptoms suggest diabetes, the consultation should not finish until a diagnosis has been made or diabetes ruled out. Children should not wait for a fasting blood glucose test. The capillary blood glucose results will be confirmed with a laboratory testing of blood glucose when the child arrives in hospital.

How is it managed?

Refer a child or young person with a high capillary blood glucose concentration promptly (same day) to secondary care for further management.

Children with type 1 diabetes require insulin, which is given in various regimens and is started on the day of referral. The management, education, and support are carried out by a multidisciplinary team based in secondary care, consisting of doctors, diabetes specialist nurses, and dietitians. Many centres are starting to use multiple injection regimens in most age groups (using basal and rapid insulin four to six times daily). Other possible regimens are two or three injections per day of various combinations of insulin types. Educating the child and family is the keystone of management, as families will need rapidly to learn

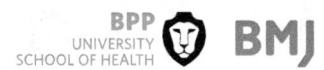

all of the practical techniques required to give insulin injections, measure blood glucose, and treat mild hypoglycaemia. Most centres admit children to hospital for up to 48 hours, but some have the resources to send children home on the first night, with follow-up and education at home.

An aggressive and relatively inexpensive campaign of information aimed at health professionals and the public on the early symptoms of diabetes dramatically reduced the incidence of diabetic ketoacidosis at diagnosis of type 1 diabetes in children in Italy.[10] A similar campaign should be tried in the UK.

Contributors: AH and JAE conceived the article; JAE and KA provided the background content about type 1 diabetes and its presentation and treatment, and AH provided the general practice perspective. All authors have provided input in the drafts. JAE is the guarantor.

Funding: No special funding.

Competing interests: All authors have completed the Unified Competing Interest form at www.icmje. org/coi_disclosure.pdf (available on request from the corresponding author) and declare: no support from any organisation for the submitted work; no financial relationships with any organisations that might have an interest in the submitted work in the previous three years, no other relationships or activities that could appear to have influenced the submitted work.

Provenance and peer review: Not commissioned, externally peer reviewed.

Patient consent not required (patient hypothetical).

1   Royal College of Paediatrics and Child Health. Growing up with diabetes: children and young people with diabetes in England. Research report. London: The College, 2009. www.rcpch.ac.uk/doc. aspx?id_Resource=4845
2   Patterson CC, Dahlquist GG, Gyürüs E, Green A, Soltész G, EURODIAB Study Group. Incidence trends for childhood type 1 diabetes in Europe during 1989-2008 and predicted new cases 2005-2020: a multicentre prospective registration study. *Lancet* 2009;373:2027-33.
3   Ali K, Wilson IV, Edge JA, Bingley PJ. Diabetic ketoacidosis at diagnosis has not declined in children over the last 20 years: data from the Bart's-Oxford Study. *Diabetic Medicine* 2009;26(suppl 1):34.
4   Pinkney JH, Bingley PJ, Sawtell PA, Dunger DB, Gale EA. Presentation and progress of childhood diabetes mellitus: a prospective population-based study. *Diabetologia* 1994;37:70-4.
5   Bui H, To T, Stein R,Fung K, Daneman D. Is diabetic ketoacidosis at disease onset a result of missed diagnosis? *J Pediatr* 2010;156:472-7.
6   Pawlowicz M, Birkholz D, Niedzwiecki M, Balcerska A. Difficulties or mistakes in diagnosing type 1 diabetes in children? The consequences of delayed diagnosis. *Pediatr Endocrinol Diabetes Metab* 2008;14:7-12.
7   Sundaram PC, Day E, Kirk JM. Delayed diagnosis in type 1 diabetes mellitus. *Arch Dis Child* 2009;94:151-2.
8   Edge JA, Ford-Adams ME, Dunger DB. Causes of death in children with insulin dependent diabetes 1990-1996. *Arch Dis Child* 1999;81:318-23.
9   Roche EF, Menon A, Gill D, Hoey H. Clinical presentation of type 1 diabetes. *Pediatr Diabetes* 2005;6:75-8.
10 Vanelli M, Chiari G, Ghizzoni L, Costi G, Giacalone T, Chiarelli F. Effectiveness of a prevention program for diabetic ketoacidosis in children. An 8-year study in schools and private practices. *Diabetes Care* 1999;22:7-9.

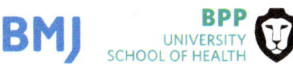

Perthes' disease

Peter Kannu, paediatrician[1], Andrew Howard, paediatric orthopaedic surgeon[2]

[1]Paediatrics, Hospital for Sick Children, Toronto, ON, Canada

[2]Orthopaedics, Hospital for Sick Children, Toronto, ON, Canada, M5G 1X8

Correspondence to: A Howard andrew.howard@sickkids.ca

Cite this as: *BMJ* 2014;349:g5584

DOI: 10.1136/bmj.g5584

www.bmj.com/content/349/bmj.g5584

A mother took her 8 year old son, who had been limping and complaining of occasional leg pain, to see their general practitioner. The boy was otherwise healthy. He walked with a limp, was afebrile, and had painful, reduced internal rotation and abduction of his right hip. Plain radiographs confirmed the diagnosis of Perthes' disease, prompting paediatric orthopaedic referral, followed by an osteotomy.

What is Perthes' disease?

Perthes' disease is the clinical manifestation of idiopathic femoral capital epiphysis vascular compromise, affecting children aged between 4 and 12 years when the epiphyseal blood supply is solely from the lateral epiphyseal vessels.[1] The annual incidence of Perthes' disease among children under the age of 15 ranges from 0.2 to 19.1 per 100 000.[2] Bilateral involvement occurs in approximately 15% of cases and is usually asymmetric. Perthes' disease affects boys three to four times more frequently than girls and is more common in children of low birth weight, children exposed to maternal smoking during pregnancy, those from lower socioeconomic groups, and children of white ethnicity.[2 3 4 5] Affected children tend to be shorter than controls and have delayed bone age.[6] Whether Perthes' disease is a single disease or the result of different pathogenetic mechanisms remains a question. A long term natural history study found that the entire clinical course of Perthes' disease lasted, on average, approximately 34 months during childhood, with long term sequelae affecting patients later in adult life.[7]

Why is Perthes' disease missed?

Musculoskeletal complaints are common in children; most are related to self resolving trauma.[8] Most have a benign clinical course requiring no specific treatment. Among many children with a painful or painless limp, however, will be a few boys and girls affected by Perthes' disease. Doctors encountering children with musculoskeletal complaints report a low confidence in their clinical skills in comparison with other body systems.[9] The medical literature suggests that just under half of cases of Perthes' disease in children are diagnosed in the advanced stages of the disease, despite pain or a limping gait being present for several months.

Why does this matter?

Untreated Perthes' disease may cause permanent femoral head deformity, followed by early onset arthritis requiring hip replacement in young adult life. Surgical treatment in early disease has been shown to improve the outcome and delay or prevent osteoarthritis for well defined subgroups of children.[10]

KEY POINTS

- Children presenting with a limp, with or without groin pain or knee pain, should be evaluated for Perthes' disease
- Physical findings include decreased hip abduction and decreased hip internal rotation compared with the unaffected side
- The diagnosis is confirmed on plain radiographs
- Early diagnosis, referral, and operative management can improve the shape of the femoral head and delay the onset of degenerative arthritis

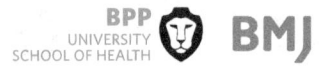

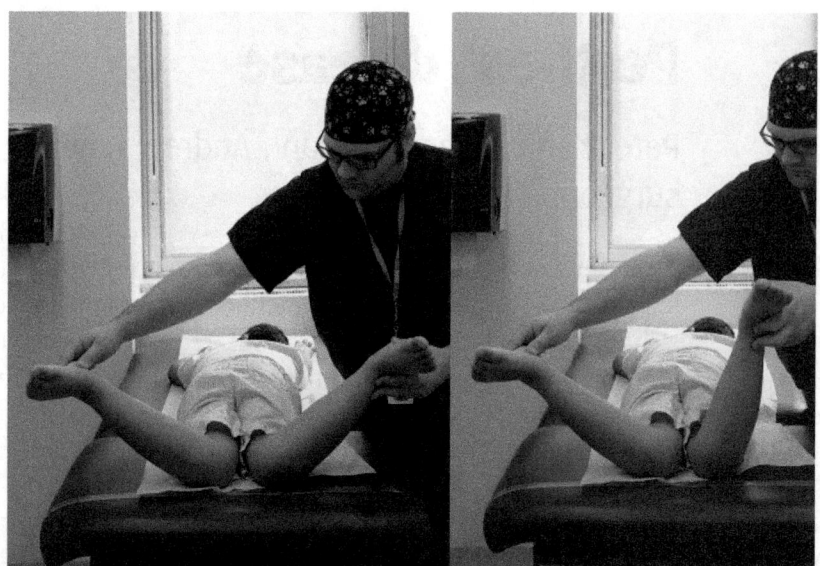

Fig 1 Examining the hips. Left: patient is prone on examining table with hips in extension; here we see symmetrical maximum internal rotation of hips. Right: a common early finding in Perthes' disease is restriction of internal rotation range, as shown on right hip here

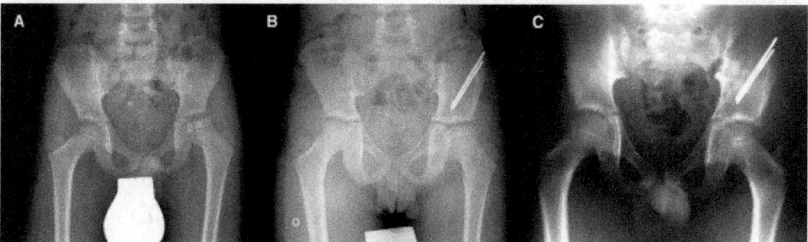

Fig 2 Radiographic findings and course of treatment. Left: radiograph of 7 year old boy with Perthes' disease showing increased density of left femoral head, with early collapse and fragmentation (right side is normal). Centre: same boy at age 9, following surgical treatment with pelvic osteotomy; femoral head is reossifying and restoring its shape. Right: the same boy at age 12, with nearly full anatomic restoration of shape of femoral head

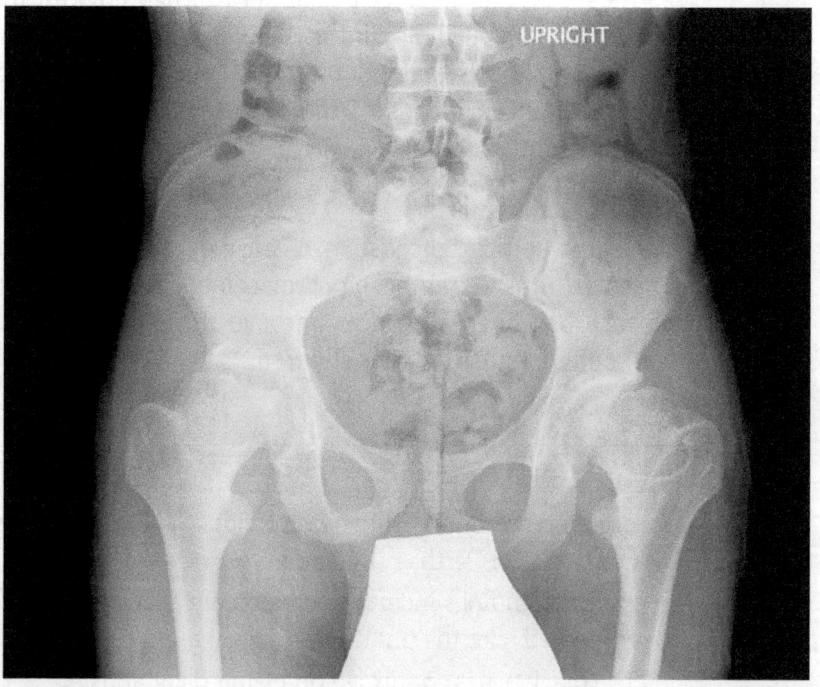

Fig 3 Radiograph of 15 year old patient who had bilateral Perthes' disease in late childhood. Femoral heads remain flattened and aspherical. Early osteoarthritis may result

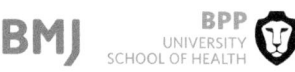

How is Perthes' disease diagnosed?

Clinical

Perthes' disease is diagnosed by characteristic changes on plain radiographs in the context of a corresponding clinical presentation. An affected child may present because of an insidious onset of a limp with or without pain. Pain may be felt at the hip (groin) but is commonly referred to the knee at this age. The child may walk with a limp. Muscle wasting in the thigh or buttock may accompany decreased abduction and internal rotation of the affected hip. We examine hip abduction with the child supine and the hips in extension, making sure the pelvis is stabilised to isolate true hip joint motion and compare one side with the other. Lying the child prone with extended hips and flexed knees allows easy comparison of internal rotation range (fig 1, left). A loss of internal rotation with or without pain at the end range is often the most sensitive clinical finding (fig 1, right).

Investigations

A full blood count together with either a C reactive protein concentration or an erythrocyte sedimentation rate is useful in excluding an inflammatory condition such as septic arthritis. A transient synovitis of the hip secondary to an intercurrent viral illness is common in children of this age group and may mimic Perthes' disease. Because the natural history of a transient synovitis is one of complete improvement over time, a child who continues to limp on follow-up should undergo repeat plain film imaging of the hips after 8-12 weeks. Anteroposterior and frog lateral radiographs of both hips are sufficient to confirm the diagnosis in most cases but occasionally may be normal in the early stages of disease. The characteristic radiological changes occur first in the femoral epiphysis and metaphysis and later in the acetabulum (fig 2, left). Plain film radiology is used to divide disease progression into four stages, each lasting several months. The first radiological stage is recognised as a dense and sclerotic femoral epiphysis. Next, the epiphysis loses height and fragments, followed by a regeneration stage and, finally, a stage of repair.

How is Perthes' disease treated?

The mainstay of management of Perthes' disease is to minimise pain, maximise motion, and avoid an irreversible femoral head deformity. Prognosis differs according to the patient's age and the stage and extent of disease. Extrusion of the femoral head occurs during the fragmentation stage of active disease and is a recognised risk factor for development of early osteoarthritis. Younger children (5-7 years old) identified at an earlier disease stage are generally treated non-operatively,[11] with range of motion exercises or activity modification encouraging swimming or cycling and discouraging vigorous jumping and landing activities. The choice of either surgical or non-surgical treatment is difficult. Experts recommend surgical treatment for children over the age of 8 and radiological staging of more advanced disease, because a prospective multicentre cohort study (with each centre applying its preferred treatment) found that operative management (osteotomy of the femur or pelvis) improved the sphericity of the femoral head at maturity compared with non-operative management with physiotherapy and/or abduction bracing.[12] Other consecutive case series have found that the use of an A-frame orthosis resulted in a high proportion of spherically congruent hips for children of all ages irrespective of the extent of disease.[13] Pain, arthritis, and ongoing hip dysfunction remain common long term sequelae in patients who are older at disease onset or who present with a poorer prognosis on the basis of radiological staging (fig 3). Studies are in progress to compare the outcomes of non-surgical and surgical treatments in 6-8 year olds and of differential surgical procedures for children over 11 years, as well as evaluating the role of drugs that limit bone resorption and potentially preserve femoral head shape.

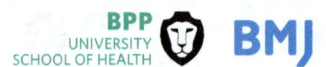

Contributors: Both authors contributed to the concept, literature review, and drafting and editing of the manuscript.

Competing interests: We have read and understood The BMJ policy on declaration of interests and declare the following interests: none.

Provenance and peer review: Commissioned; externally peer reviewed.

Patient consent obtained.

1 Chung SM. The arterial supply of the developing proximal end of the human femur. *J Bone Joint Surg Am* 1976;58:961-70.

2 Perry DC, Machin DM, Pope D, Bruce CE, Dangerfield P, Platt MJ, et al. Racial and geographic factors in the incidence of Legg-Calve-Perthes' disease: a systematic review. *Am J Epidemiol* 2012;175:159-66.

3 Kim HK. Legg-Calve-Perthes disease: etiology, pathogenesis, and biology. *J Pediatr Orthop* 2011;31(2 suppl):S141-6.

4 Hall AJ, Barker DJ, Dangerfield PH, Taylor JF. Perthes' disease of the hip in Liverpool. *Br Med J (Clin Res Ed)* 1983;287:1757-9.

5 Bahmanyar S, Montgomery SM, Weiss RJ, Ekbom A. Maternal smoking during pregnancy, other prenatal and perinatal factors, and the risk of Legg-Calve-Perthes disease. *Pediatrics* 2008;122:e459-64.

6 Lee ST, Vaidya SV, Song HR, Lee SH, Suh SW, Telang SS. Bone age delay patterns in Legg-Calve-Perthes disease: an analysis using the Tanner and Whitehouse 3 method. *J Pediatr Orthop* 2007;27:198-203.

7 Joseph B, Varghese G, Mulpuri K, Narasimha Rao K, Nair NS. Natural evolution of Perthes disease: a study of 610 children under 12 years of age at disease onset. *J Pediatr Orthop* 2003;23:590-600.

8 De Inocencio J. Epidemiology of musculoskeletal pain in primary care. *Arch Dis Child* 2004;89:431-4.

9 Jandial S, Myers A, Wise E, Foster HE. Doctors likely to encounter children with musculoskeletal complaints have low confidence in their clinical skills. *J Pediatr* 2009;154:267-71.

10 Wiig O, Terjesen T, Svenningsen S. Prognostic factors and outcome of treatment in Perthes' disease: a prospective study of 368 patients with five-year follow-up. *J Bone Joint Surg Br* 2008;90:1364-71.

11 Nguyen NA, Klein G, Dogbey G, McCourt JB, Mehlman CT. Operative versus nonoperative treatments for Legg-Calve-Perthes disease: a meta-analysis. *J Pediatr Orthop* 2012;32:697-705.

12 Herring JA. Legg-Calve-Perthes disease at 100: a review of evidence-based treatment. *J Pediatr Orthop* 2011;31(2 suppl):S137-40.

13 Rich MM, Schoenecker PL. Management of Legg-Calve-Perthes disease using an A-frame orthosis and hip range of motion: a 25-year experience. *J Pediatr Orthop* 2013;33:112-9.

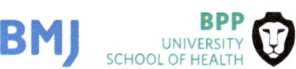

Slipped capital femoral epiphysis

N M P Clarke, consultant orthopaedic surgeon,
Tony Kendrick, associate dean for clinical research, professor of primary medical care

Southampton University Hospitals NHS Trust, Southampton General Hospital, Southampton SO16 6YD

Correspondence to: N M P Clarke ortho@soton.ac.uk

Cite this as: *BMJ* 2009;339:b4457

DOI: 10.1136/bmj.b4457

www.bmj.com/ content/339/bmj.b4457

Slipped capital (or upper) femoral epiphysis occurs during periods of rapid growth in adolescence, when shear forces, particularly in obese children, increase across the proximal femoral growth plate, leading to displacement of the epiphysis. The typical patient is obese. In a recent case study of 54 patients with this condition, all had body mass indexes in the overweight or obese ranges.[1] In boys, accompanying hypogonadism implicates possible endocrine causes.[2] A chronic slip is the most common presentation, with symptoms present for weeks or months as the slip progresses. An acute slip occurs after a traumatic event and prevents weight bearing, whereas in an acute on chronic slip, prodromal symptoms are followed by a sudden exacerbation of pain. The last two types of slip usually present to the emergency department rather than the general practitioner.

Why is it missed?

The indolent nature of the symptoms in a chronic slip and pain referred to the knee often mislead the doctor. Examination of the hip may be overlooked and the diagnosis missed. In a review of 106 patients, those (n=14) who had pain in the knee or distal thigh only were more likely to be misdiagnosed, have unnecessary radiographs, and have more severe slips on confirmation of the diagnosis.[5]

Why does this matter?

Chronic slippage will gradually progress in terms of severity of displacement and deformity, with increasing limb shortening and external rotation, as confirmed by a recent case series.[6] Alternatively, after prodromal symptoms, sudden severe pain may occur with minor trauma such as a fall. This indicates an acute on chronic slip, with major epiphyseal displacement and an increased risk of ischaemic injury and avascular necrosis, which can have devastating consequences. Major surgery may also be needed. Residual deformity causes femoroacetabular impingement and premature osteoarthritis.[7]

How is it diagnosed?

Clinical features

Any child or adolescent who presents with knee pain must undergo careful examination of the hip. Loss of internal rotation of the leg in flexion, with pain at the extreme of movement, is the key physical sign.

Investigations

Anteroposterior and lateral radiographs of both hips on the same film are the primary (and usually the only) imaging needed to diagnose and evaluate the condition. Klein's line drawn parallel to the superior neck on the anteroposterior view will normally intersect the lateral

---

KEY POINTS

- Knee pain in adolescents should trigger a careful examination of the hip because it may be caused by slipped capital (or upper) femoral epiphysis
- Delayed diagnosis is associated with an increased slip and hence deformity and morbidity
- Radiography in anteroposterior and lateral planes confirms the diagnosis
- Surgical treatment of an early slip leads to an almost normal outcome

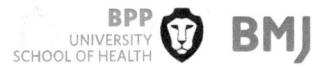

portion of the femoral epiphysis but not if slipped (Trethowan's sign; fig 1).[8] Slipped capital femoral epiphysis must be excluded before investigation for other pathology.

HOW COMMON IS IT?

- Incidence is 1-7 per 100 000
- It is three times more common in boys than in girls
- A bilateral slip occurs in about 20% of cases[3]
- Delayed diagnosis is common. One review of 102 patients reported a mean delay of 2.5 months and apparent initial misdiagnosis in 52% of cases[4]

CASE SCENARIO

A 13 year old boy visited the general practitioner because of a six week history of intermittent limp and pain in the left lower thigh and knee, which was exacerbated by playing sports. On examination he was overweight, but he had no abnormality in the knee. "Knee strain" was diagnosed, and he was advised to take ibuprofen and abstain from sports. Four weeks later he returned with worsening more persistent pain, now in the thigh as well as the knee. Careful examination of the hip elicited a degree of restriction of flexion and rotation, both internal and external, with 2 cm shortening of the affected leg. Radiography of the left hip showed a slipped capital femoral epiphysis.

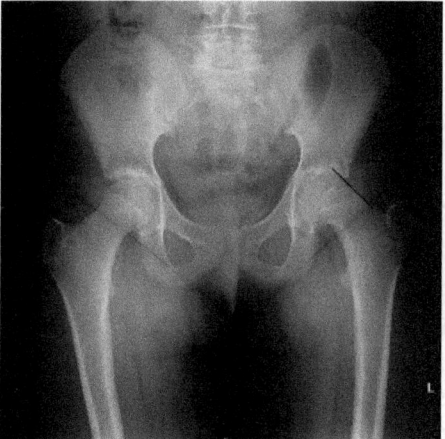

Fig 1 Anteroposterior radiograph of the hips and pelvis showing a minor left slipped capital femoral epiphysis. Klein's line drawn along the superior femoral neck does not intersect the lateral portion of the epiphysis

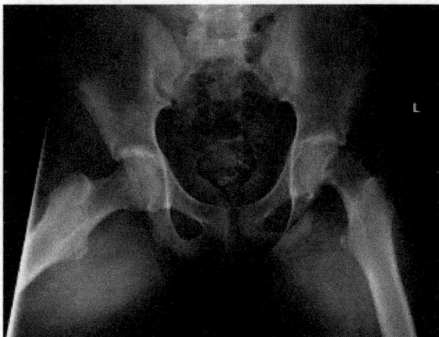

Fig 2 The same patient two weeks later, after an exacerbation of pain. The radiograph shows increased slip of the left capital femoral epiphysis, with further displacement

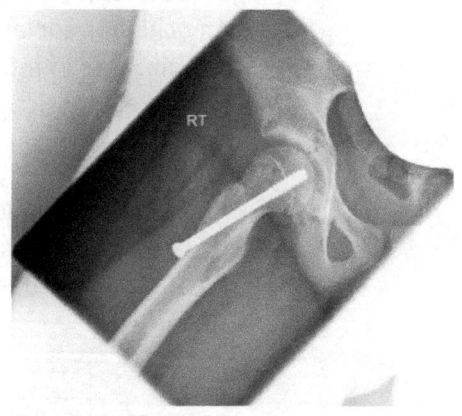

Fig 3 Screw fixation

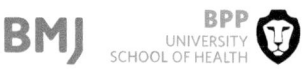

How is it managed?

Once the diagnosis has been confirmed the usual treatment—based on expert consensus and experience—is to admit the patient urgently to hospital and place on bed rest to avoid acute displacement of a chronic slip, which can have a catastrophic affect on prognosis (fig 2).[9] Surgery is needed to stabilise a displaced capital femoral epiphysis and prevent further displacement and increasing deformity. This is achieved by single cannulated screw fixation under image intensifier control (fig 3). The more severe the deformity the more challenging the procedure, necessitating different entry points. Very severe displacement may necessitate femoral neck osteotomy or subsequent salvage procedures for persistent deformity. Remodelling can occur in younger patients.[10] Avascular necrosis and chondrolysis (chemical necrosis of articular cartilage) are the most common complications, the first usually after acute displacement (up to 35% of cases), but both may occur after surgery. Reports of the incidence of chrondrolysis after screw fixation vary, but some are as low as 1.5%.[11]

Contributors: NMPC was the main author of this article and TK contributed. NMPC is guarantor.

Funding: No special funding received.

Competing interests: None declared.

Provenance and peer review: Not commissioned; externally peer reviewed.

Patient consent not required (patient anonymised, dead, or hypothetical).

1   Bhatia NN, Pirpiris M, Otsuka NY. Body mass index in patients with slipped capital femoral epiphysis. *J Pediatr Orthop* 2006;26:197-9.
2   Aronsson DD, Loder RT, Breur GJ, Weinstein SL. Slipped capital femoral epiphysis: current concepts. *J Am Acad Orthop Surg* 2006;14:666-79.
3   Lehmann CL, Arons RR, Loder RT, Vitale MG. The epidemiology of slipped capital femoral epiphysis: an update. *J Pediatr Orthop* 2006;26:286-9.
4   Green DW, Reynolds RA, Khan SN, Tolo V. The delay in diagnosis of slipped capital femoral epiphysis: a review of 102 patients. *HSS J* 2005;1:103-6.
5   Matava MJ, Patton CM, Luhmann S, Gordon JE, Schoenecker PL. Knee pain as the initial symptom of slipped capital femoral epiphysis: an analysis of initial presentation and treatment. *J Pediatr Orthop* 1999;19:455-60.
6   Rahme D, Comley A, Foster B, Cundy P. Consequences of diagnostic delays in slipped capital femoral epiphysis. *J Pediatr Orthop B* 2006;15:93-7.
7   Carney BT, Weinstein SL, Noble J. Long term follow up of slipped capital femoral epiphysis. *J Bone Joint Surg Am* 1991;73:667-74.
8   Klein A, Joplin RJ, Reidy JA, Hanelin J. Roentgenographic fractures of slipped capital femoral epiphysis. *Am J Roentgenol Radium Ther* 1951;66:361-74.
9   Kallio PE, Mah ET, Foster BK, Paterson DC, LeQuesne GW. Slipped capital femoral epiphysis: incidence and clinical assessment of physeal instability. *J Bone Joint Surg Br* 1995;77:752-5.
10 Jones JR, Paterson DC, Hillier TM, Foster BK, Remodelling after pinning for slipped capital femoral epiphysis. *J Bone Joint Surg Br* 1990;72:568-73.
11 Loder RT. Slipped capital femoral epiphysis. In: Staheli LT, Song KM, eds. Pediatric orthopaedic secrets. Mosby, 2007:353-8.

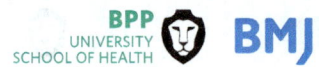

Testicular torsion

Bhaskar K Somani, specialist registrar in urology[1],
Graham Watson, general practitioner[2],
Nick Townell, consultant urological surgeon[1]

[1]Ninewells Hospital, Dundee DD1 9SY

[2]Dundee

Correspondence to: N Townell nicktownell@nhs.net

Cite this as: *BMJ* 2010;341:c3213

DOI: 10.1136/bmj.c3213

www.bmj.com/content/341/bmj.c3213

Testicular torsion is a surgical emergency requiring prompt diagnosis and specialist referral. In all cases of suspected testicular torsion, emergency surgical exploration is necessary to avoid loss of the testicle.

How common is it?

Testicular torsion has a bimodal age distribution, occurring either soon after birth or more commonly at puberty, but it can occur in any age group. The annual incidence in males <25 years is 1 in 4000.[1] The incidence of testicular torsion, torsion of testicular appendage, and epididymitis was 16%, 46%, and 35%, respectively, in 238 children presenting with acute scrotal pain.[2] In a prospective audit of 173 scrotal explorations for suspected testicular torsion over an 11 year period (1998-2008) in our centre, 89 (51%) had testicular torsion and 16 (9%) required an orchidectomy due to delayed presentation, with 75% (12) presenting 24 hours or more after onset of symptoms.[3] When general practitioners were aware of possible testicular torsion and thus referred patients as soon as possible, the orchidectomy rate was lower than in patients who presented later and whose referral was delayed.[4 5]

Why is it missed?

Testicular pain and tenderness may be absent in up to a third of the patients.[6] Swelling of the testis or scrotum, oedema or erythema of scrotal skin, and abdominal pain may be the presenting symptom in these cases. Pain may be intermittent (with episodes of torsion and detorsion) or a dull ache of gradual onset; it may also be referred to abdominal or inguinoscrotal regions. In a screaming male infant, the scrotum may not always be carefully examined to exclude a torsion, as this diagnosis may be overlooked as a cause for infant distress.

Why does this matter?

Torsion may lead to testicular ischaemia, with eventual haemorrhagic infarction and testicular necrosis.[7] Ischaemic changes can begin within hours, and complete testicular atrophy will ensue in most cases after 24 hours[8] unless surgical exploration results in manual detorsion. Detorsion within six hours of onset of symptoms has a salvage rate of 90-100%, which drops to 20-50% after 12 hours and to 10% after 24 hours.[9] Normal sperm counts occur in only 5-50% of patients after orchidectomy or if testicular atrophy develops.[10]

KEY POINTS

- Testicular torsion may be difficult to diagnose if symptoms are intermittent or atypical, but it must be considered in all cases of scrotal pain, with careful history and examination
- Sudden, severe onset of testicular pain with tenderness should be considered as torsion and referred, unless other clinical features suggest an alternative diagnosis
- Examine the testis for tenderness, size, shape, and position, and examine the remaining scrotal contents, comparing findings with the unaffected side
- A colour duplex ultrasound scan may be very accurate if intratesticular blood flow is absent, but findings may not be diagnostic in early or intermittent torsion
- Urgent scrotal exploration and bilateral testicular fixation should be performed in all cases of suspected testicular torsion

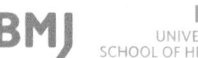

> **CASE SCENARIO**
>
> A 17 year old man presented with a 24 hour history of intermittent testicular pain without any urinary symptoms. The testis was mildly tender with no swelling and felt normal in size, shape, and position. A diagnosis of possible orchitis was made, but he was referred for further assessment. Surgical exploration found an engorged testis, confirming a diagnosis of intermittent torsion.

How is it diagnosed?

Clinical features

Several case series describe the clinical features associated with testicular torsion, but exact prevalence is difficult to ascertain.[6] [11] [12] Testicular pain occurs in 70-90% of cases, testicular or scrotal oedema in 60-75% of cases, abdominal pain in 7-28% of cases, and nausea or vomiting in 5-43% of cases.

Characteristically, testicular pain is of sudden and severe onset; it may radiate to the groin or lower abdomen and be accompanied by nausea, vomiting, and fever. Excluding a history of any other lower urinary tract symptoms such as frequency, urgency, or dysuria and taking a relevant social and sexual history can help exclude genitourinary infection as a cause of the symptoms.

Physical examination should include genital, inguinal, and abdominal examinations. Testicular examination should be done for lie (high or low) and axis (horizontal or vertical), comparing the affected to the unaffected side. Tender, elevated, transversely located testis with loss of cremasteric reflex suggests testicular torsion.[12]

Investigations

Urinalysis positive for nitrite and leucocyte esterase may indicate a urinary tract infection, although if a clinical suspicion of testicular torsion persists, the patient should be referred for specialist assessment. Colour duplex scrotal ultrasound may be useful. Absence of intratesticular blood flow was 86% sensitive, 100% specific, and 97% accurate in the diagnosis in one study,[13] although accuracy rates are operator dependent, and peripheral flow may be present in early torsion or with episodes of torsion and detorsion. Hence, the decision to surgically explore should be made on clinical grounds. In our case scenario, intermittent testicular torsion was diagnosed from clinical history. Surgery in such cases results in resolution of pain and prevents future testicular infarction.[14]

How is it managed?

All clinically obvious cases of testicular torsion, or those diagnosed with colour duplex ultrasonography, should be treated as an emergency.[15] Scrotal exploration with detorsion of the affected side and bilateral testicular fixation should be performed.[16] Ideally a three point fixation of the testis within the scrotum prevents further torsion. Patients should also be warned about an orchidectomy if the testis cannot be salvaged.

Contributors: BKS wrote the first draft of the article, which was modified by GW and NT. The final draft was agreed with NT. NT is the guarantor for the paper.

Funding: No external funding.

Competing interests: None declared.

Patient consent not required (patient anonymised, dead, or hypothetical).

Provenance and peer review: Commissioned; externally peer reviewed.

1   Barada JH, Weingarten JL, Cromie WJ. Testicular salvage and age-related delay in the presentation of testicular torsion. *J Urol* 1989;142:746-8.
2   Lewis AG, Bukowski TP, Jarvis PD, Wacksman J, Sheldon CA. Evaluation of acute scrotum in the emergency department. *Pediatr Surg* 1995;30:277-81.
3   Molokwu CN, Somani BK, Goodman CM. Surgical outcome of exploration for acute scrotal pain: a consecutive case series of 173 patients. *BJU Int* 2010 (in press).
4   Anderson JB, Williamson RC. Testicular torsion in Bristol: a 25-year review. *Br J Surg* 1988;75:988-92.

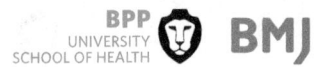

5   Bennett S, Nicholson MS, Little TM. Torsion of the testis: why is the prognosis so poor? *BMJ* 1987;294:824.

6   Mäkelä E, Lahdes-Vasama T, Rajakorpi H, Wikström S. A 19-year review of paediatric patients with acute scrotum. *Scand J Surg* 2007;96:62-6.

7   Smith GI. Cellular changes from graded testicular ischemia. *J Urol* 1955;73:355-62.

8   Visser AJ, Heyns CF. Testicular function after torsion of the spermatic cord. *BJU Int* 2003;92:200-3.

9   Cattolica EV, Karol JB, Rankin KN, Klein RS. High testicular salvage rate in torsion of the spermatic cord. *J Urol* 1982;128:66-8.

10 Brasso K, Andersen L, Kay L, Wille-Jørgensen P, Linnet L, Egense J. Testicular torsion: a follow-up study. *Scand J Urol Nephrol* 1993;27:1-6.

11 Mushtaq I, Fung M, Glasson MJ. Retrospective review of paediatric patients with acute scrotum. *Aust N Z J Surg* 2003;73:55-8.

12 Ciftci AO, Senocak ME, Tanyel FC, Büyükpamukçu N. Clinical predictors for differential diagnosis of acute scrotum. *Eur J Pediatr Surg* 2004;14:333-8.

13 Burks DD, Markey BJ, Burkhard TK, Balsara ZN, Haluszka MM, Canning DA. Suspected testicular torsion and ischemia: evaluation with color Doppler sonography. *Radiology* 1990;175:815-21.

14 Eaton SH, Cendron MA, Estrada CR, Bauer SB, Borer JG, Cilento BG, et al. Intermittent testicular torsion: diagnostic features and management outcomes. *J Urol* 2005;174:1532-5.

15 Jefferson RH, Perez LM, Joseph DB. Critical analysis of the clinical presentation of acute scrotum: a 9-year experience at a single institution. *J Urol* 1997;158:1198-200.

16 Sessions AE, Rabinowitz R, Hulbert WC, Goldstein MM, Mevorach RA. Testicular torsion: direction, degree, duration and disinformation. *J Urol* 2003;169:663-5.

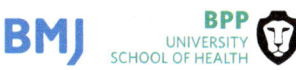

Long QT syndrome

Dominic J Abrams, consultant cardiologist and electrophysiologist[1],
Malcolm A Perkin, general practitioner[2],
Jonathan R Skinner, consultant paediatric cardiologist and electrophysiologist[3]

[1]Department of Cardiac Electrophysiology, St Bartholomew's Hospital and Great Ormond Street Hospital for Children, London

[2]Roysia Surgery, Royston

[3]Green Lane Paediatric and Congenital Cardiac Services, Starship Children's Hospital, Auckland, New Zealand

Correspondence to: Dr D J Abrams, Department of Cardiac Electrophysiology, St Bartholomew's Hospital, London EC1A 7BE
d.abrams@qmul.ac.uk

Cite this as: *BMJ* 2010;340:b4815

DOI: 10.1136/bmj.b4815

www.bmj.com/content/340/bmj.b4815

Congenital long QT syndrome is a potential cause of avoidable sudden cardiac death. Affected individuals may have ventricular arrhythmias, leading to palpitations, syncope, and, if sustained, cardiac arrest.[1] The syndrome is inherited in an autosomal dominant fashion, with variable disease expression: those severely affected may die in fetal or neonatal life, but others remain asymptomatic throughout their life. At a cellular level, genetically encoded abnormalities in sodium and potassium ion channels within the cell membrane lengthen cardiac repolarisation, which manifests as a prolongation of the QT interval in the electrocardiogram. QT prolongation may be acquired secondary to certain medications, metabolic disturbance, cerebral injury, myocardial disease, and hypothermia—factors that may also unmask the congenital syndrome in a previously asymptomatic individual.

Why is long QT syndrome missed?

Syncope is highly prevalent in young adults. Among 394 students, 154 reported at least one episode of syncope.[4] In a young, fit adult (such as outlined in the scenario box), important differential diagnoses include the most common and benign cause of syncope, neurocardiogenic (vasovagal) syncope,[4] as well as primary arrhythmias, cardiomyopathies, and structural heart disease that all warrant further cardiology evaluation. Cerebral hypoperfusion during arrhythmic syncope may manifest as myoclonic jerks or epileptic type movements,[5] leading to long QT syndrome often being misdiagnosed as epilepsy. In a recent study 39% of patients in a cohort with long QT syndrome had a delayed diagnosis after presentation with seizures or syncope, which were most frequently misdiagnosed as epilepsy but also as breath-holding attacks and vasovagal syncope. The time between presentation and diagnosis of long QT syndrome ranged from two months to 23 years, and in four cases another family member died before the correct diagnosis had been made.[6]

Why does this matter?

In long QT syndrome, prolongation of the QT interval and appropriately timed ventricular ectopy (R on T phenomenon) leads to the development of torsades de pointes, a ventricular arrhythmia with a classic appearance in an electrocardiogram (figure 1). Torsades de pointes will often resolve spontaneously, although may degenerate to ventricular fibrillation, leading to cardiac arrest and potentially sudden cardiac death. Early identification of a patient with long QT syndrome and prompt, appropriate treatment are therefore critical to prevent cardiac

---

KEY POINTS

- Long QT syndrome is a familial condition associated with recurrent syncope and sudden cardiac death resulting from ventricular arrhythmias; it may be misdiagnosed as epilepsy
- Triggers for arrhythmias may include medications that prolong the QT interval or subtype specific factors such as swimming and other exercise (long QT1), auditory stimuli and emotional stress (long QT2), and rest or sleep (long QT3)
- β blockers are usually highly effective, with implantable cardioverter defibrillators reserved for people deemed at high risk or refractory to medical treatment
- Thoracoscopic left cardiac sympathectomy is highly effective and is useful if β blockers are not tolerated or an implantable cardioverter defibrillator is contraindicated

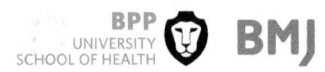

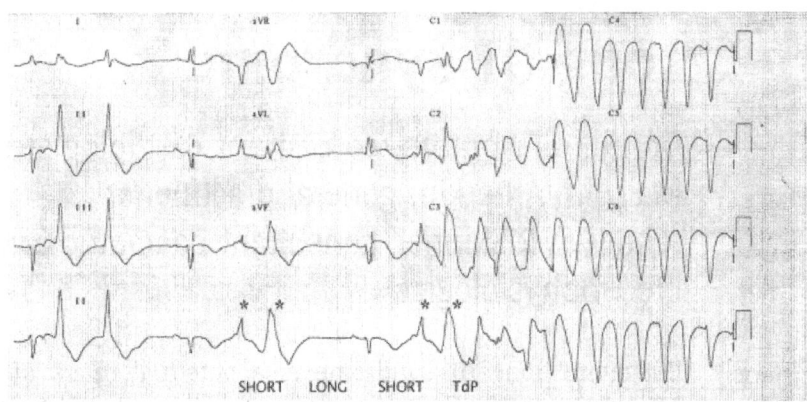

SHORT LONG SHORT TdP

Fig 1 Initiation of torsades de pointes. A 12 lead electrocardiogram and rhythm strip (lead II) recorded from a patient with long QT syndrome and a corrected QT interval of 540 ms. The rhythm strip at the bottom of the image shows numerous ventricular extrasystoles (indicated by asterisks) creating alternating short, long, and short RR intervals initiating torsades de pointes (TdP)

CASE SCENARIO

A 19 year old female student consulted her general practitioner about two recent episodes of syncope, both of which occurred while playing hockey. Her team mates reported that she collapsed suddenly with little warning, recovering rapidly within 30 seconds without confusion. She was otherwise well, although she was taking erythromycin for an infected leg abrasion at the time of the events. As part of the routine evaluation for syncope, her general practitioner performed a 12 lead electrocardiogram, which showed a prolonged corrected QT interval of 510 ms.

HOW COMMON IS LONG QT SYNDROME?

- The exact prevalence of long QT syndrome in the population is unknown as disease expression may be highly variable

- Current population estimates range from 1 in 2000[2] to 1 in 3000[3]

- Most general practices in the UK are likely therefore to have at least one patient with the condition

---

events. All drugs that prolong the QT interval should be stringently avoided in patients with long QT syndrome (box). As the syndrome is an inherited condition, identification of other family members at risk is essential.

How is it diagnosed?

The diagnosis is a clinical one based on electrocardiographic findings and clinical and family history.

Clinical features

History taking

An accurate history is essential, so ask patients to talk through the event(s) step by step, carefully describing their symptoms and timing. Seek witness statements where possible. Features that stand out are listed below.

- *Exertional syncope*—this should always raise alarm of a sinister cause. Three genetically and clinically distinct subtypes of congenital long QT syndrome exist:

- Long QT1 is associated with events during exercise, particularly swimming, with frequent symptoms but lower mortality

- Long QT2 events occur during emotional stress or auditory stimuli, especially waking from sleep (such as ringing telephones and alarm clocks)

- Long QT3 is associated with events at rest; such events are less common but have a higher associated mortality.[1]

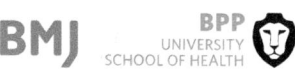

COMMONLY PRESCRIBED AGENTS THAT PROLONG QT INTERVAL AND SHOULD BE AVOIDED IN PATIENTS WITH CONGENITAL LONG QT SYNDROME*

Antiarrhythmics
- Amiodarone
- Sotalol

Antibiotics
- Erythromycin
- Clarithromycin
- Ciprofloxacin

Antihistamines
- Terfenadine

Antidepressants
- Fluoxetine
- Sertraline
- Amitryptiline

*A comprehensive list is available at www.azcert.org

- *Vasovagal syncope*—this is most commonly triggered by a warm environment, prolonged standing, painful stimuli, or insufficient food intake.[4]

- *Sudden syncopal events*—as in the case scenario we describe, these are an atypical feature of vasovagal syncope, in which dizziness, sweating, and visual disturbances often precede loss of consciousness. In long QT syndrome patients may have rapid palpitations as the first symptom, whereas a compensatory sinus tachycardia after the onset of other symptoms may occur in benign syncope.

- *Rapid recovery*—after the syncopal event, rapid recovery without confusion or drowsiness is characteristic of cardiac syncope. Although epileptic-type movements secondary to cerebral anoxia may occur in long QT syndrome,[5][6] neurological features such as aura and postictal confusion are typically absent.

- *Drug history*—ask about any drugs used when symptoms were present as many commonly used agents (box) prolong the QT interval and may precipitate cardiac arrhythmias in patients with long QT syndrome.[7] Similarly, unexplained syncope in older patients should trigger a careful review of medication.

- *Family history*—ask specifically whether there is a family history of unexplained sudden death (including in young children), refractory epilepsy, or recurrent syncope.

Clinical examination
Patients with long QT syndrome have a structurally and functionally normal heart, so a cardiac examination will yield a normal result. Any abnormal findings on cardiac examination suggest a structural or cardiomyopathic cause of syncope instead.

Investigations
Measurement of the QT interval in the electrocardiogram is the primary investigation, with figures of >450 ms in males and >460 ms in females suggesting QT prolongation. The QT interval is calculated automatically and displayed on the electrocardiogram, but errors are common, and manual measurement is advised (figure 2). Inaccurate calculation of the QT interval[2] may lead to a false negative[6] or false positive diagnosis.[8] Measurement of the QT interval after exercise testing[9] or at times of bradycardia on 24 hour Holter monitoring may help in the identification of carriers of the long QT gene who have a normal QT interval on resting electrocardiographic evaluation.

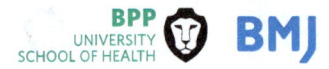

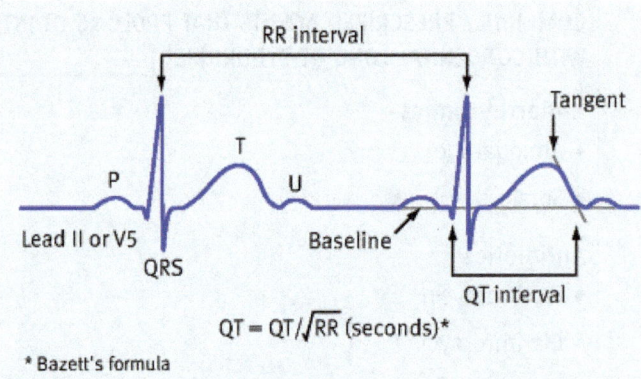

$$QT = QT/\sqrt{RR} \text{ (seconds)}*$$

* Bazett's formula

Fig 2 Measurement of the QT interval using the tangent technique. The QT interval is measured from the onset of the Q wave to the end of the T wave, defined as the intersection of the tangent to the steepest downslope of the T wave and the baseline. To adjust for the effects of heart rate, Bazett's formula is used to calculate the corrected QT interval (QTc) Adapted with permission from Postema et al[2]

Once long QT syndrome has been diagnosed definitively, genetic analysis for mutations in the genes encoding for cardiac ion channels may be helpful in confirming the subtype and in identifying all other affected family members. At present 65-70% of affected individuals will have an identifiable mutation in the known genes.

How is it managed?

The mainstay of treatment is β blockers. These are most effective in the long QT1 subtype, in which the prognosis is excellent if patients avoid drugs that prolong the QT interval[7] and specific triggers such as competitive exercise.[10] Although β blockers are least effective in long QT3, they may still be beneficial.[11] Patients should continue taking β blockers at all times, including pregnancy and peripartum.[12] As in any long term treatment, non-compliance[7] and contraindications (such as asthma) provide particular challenges. In high risk patients (including those who have survived a cardiac arrest, those with a recent history of syncope or with a QT interval >500 ms, males under 18 years, or females over 18 years[13 14]), consider implantable cardioverter defibrillators in conjunction with β blockers. If β blockers are not tolerated, defibrillators are contraindicated, or symptoms persist despite optimal β blockade, thoracoscopic left cardiac sympathectomy is highly effective.[15] All patients should be given a list of medications that prolong the QT interval and be advised carefully of specific triggers.

Contributors: DJA wrote the article with contributions and modifications from MAP and JRS. DJA is the guarantor for the paper.

Funding: No special finding.

Competing interests: None declared.

Provenance and peer review: Not commissioned; externally peer reviewed.

Patient consent not required (patient anonymised, dead, or hypothetical).

1 Morita H, Wu J, Zipes DP. The QT syndromes: long and short. *Lancet* 2008;372:750-63.
2 Postema PG, de Jong JSSG, van der Bilt IAC, Wilde AAM. Accurate electrocardiographic assessment of the QT interval: teach the tangent. *Heart Rhythm* 2008;5:1015-8.
3 Hayashi K, Fujino N, Uchiyama K, Ino H, Sakata K, Konno T, et al. Long QT syndrome and associated gene mutation carriers in Japanese children: results from ECG screening examination. *Clin Sci (Lond)* 2009;117:415-24.
4 Ganzeboom KS, Colman N, Reitsma JB, Shen WK, Wieling W. Prevalence and triggers of syncope in medical students. *Am J Cardiol* 2003;91:1006-8.
5 Lempert T, Bauer M, Schmidt D. Syncope: a videometric analysis of 56 episodes of transient cerebral hypoxia. *Ann Neurol* 1994;36:233-7.
6 MacCormick JM, McAlister H, Crawford J, French JK, Crozier I, Shelling AN, et al. Misdiagnosis of long QT syndrome as epilepsy at first presentation. *Ann Emerg Med* 2009;54:26-32.
7 Vincent GM, Schwartz PJ, Denjoy I, Swan H, Bithell C, Spazzolini C, et al. High efficacy of beta-blockers in long-QT syndrome type 1: contribution of noncompliance and QT-prolonging drugs to the occurrence of beta-blocker treatment "failures." *Circulation* 2009;119:215-21.

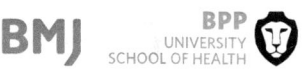

8   Taggart NW, Haglund CM, Tester DJ, Ackerman MJ. Diagnostic miscues in congenital long QT syndrome. *Circulation* 2007;115:2613-20.

9   Swann H, Viitasalo M, Piippo K, Laitinen P, Kontula K, Toivonen L. Sinus node function and ventricular reploarization during exercise stress test in long QT syndrome patients with KvLQT1 and HERG potassium channel defects. *J Am Coll Cardiol* 1999;34:823-9.

10   Maron BJ, Chaitman BR, Ackerman MJ, Bayés de Luna A, Corrado D, Crosson JE, et al. Recommendations for physical activity and recreational sports participation for young patients with genetic cardiovascular diseases. *Circulation* 2004;109:2807-16.

11   Schwartz PJ, Spazzolini C, Crotti L. All LQT3 patients need an ICD: true of false. *Heart Rhythm* 2009;6:113-20.

12   Seth R, Moss AJ, McNitt S, Zareba W, Andrews ML, Qi M, et al. Long QT syndrome and pregnancy. *J Am Coll Cardiol* 2007;49:1092-8.

13   Goldenberg I, Moss AJ, Peterson DR, McNitt S, Zareba W, Andrews ML, et al. Risk factors for aborted cardiac arrest and sudden cardiac death in children with congenital long QT syndrome. *Circulation* 2008;117:2184-91.

14   Sauer AJ, Moss AJ, McNitt S, Peterson DR, Zareba W, Robinson JL, et al. Long QT syndrome in adults. *J Am Coll Cardiol* 2007;49:329-37.

15   Schwartz PJ, Priori SG, Cerrone M, Spazzolini C, Odero A, Napolitano C, et al. Left cardiac sympathetic denervation in the management of high risk patients affected by the long QT syndrome. *Circulation* 2004;109:1826-33.

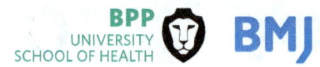

Nasal septal haematoma

Leigh N Sanyaolu, core surgical trainee (ear, nose, and throat),
Sarah E J Farmer, specialist registrar (ear, nose, and throat),
Patrick J Cuddihy, consultant (ear, nose, and throat)

Department of Otolaryngology, Royal Gwent Hospital, Newport, UK

Correspondence to: L N Sanyaolu lnsanyaolu@doctors.org.uk

Cite this as: *BMJ* 2014;349:g6075

DOI: 10.1136/bmj.g6075

www.bmj.com/content/349/bmj.g6075

A 15 year old boy attends the emergency department with his mother after sustaining a nasal injury while playing rugby. His mother is worried that her son has fractured his nose. The boy says that his nose feels "very blocked" but otherwise he feels well. Examination shows a swollen nose with some associated bruising and the suspicion of bony nasal deviation to the left. Anterior rhinoscopy shows a bilateral cherry red swelling arising from the nasal septum. An immediate referral is made to the ear, nose, and throat department and the patient undergoes an emergency operation to incise and drain a septal haematoma, with no permanent damage to the nasal septum.

What is a nasal septal haematoma?

Nasal trauma is extremely common, with the nasal bones being the third most commonly fractured bone in the human body.[1][2][3] In about 90% of nasal fractures the nasal septum is also injured.[1][2][3] A potential serious complication of nasal trauma is a nasal septal haematoma. This is the development of a haematoma between the septal cartilage and the overlying mucoperichondrium.[3][4] Damage to the septal cartilage can occur within 24 hours, and if untreated it can rapidly lead to irreversible septal destruction and substantial nasal deformity requiring extensive reconstruction.[2][5][6]

Why is a nasal septal haematoma missed?

A nasal septal haematoma can occur after minor trauma. Nasal trauma is common in children. It is hypothesised that because the septal cartilage of children is softer than that of adults, it is more likely to buckle secontdary to trauma, making the formation of haematomas more likely.[8] Also, although rare, cases of spontaneous septal haematoma have been reported.[7][9] External injury might not be obvious and symptoms can be non-specific, particularly in children, therefore a high index of suspicion is needed in any patient presenting with a history of nasal injury, however innocuous it might seem.[10]

A considerable proportion of patients with nasal injuries seen in emergency departments have no documented evidence of the nasal septum being examined and the presence of a septal haematoma being assessed.[7][11] This problem is often exacerbated by a lack of guidelines for the treatment of nasal injuries in such departments.[12] It is important that patients with nasal trauma are assessed thoroughly for the presence of a septal haematoma and that this is appropriately documented.

Why does this matter?

Untreated nasal septal haematoma can lead to irreversible septal necrosis within 72-96 hours.[6] The exact mechanism by which this occurs is debated. It is thought that trauma causes rupture of small sub-mucosal septal vessels and that blood then accumulates between the nasal septum and the mucoperichondrium to form the haematoma.[4][5] This can result in pressure related ischaemia of the cartilage and subsequent necrosis of the septal cartilage.[4][5]

Once septal necrosis has occurred the structural integrity of the nose can be disrupted and the dorsum of the nose affected, leading to severe cosmetic distortion of the nose. In a case series of seven patients, all developed sequelae, with most developing substantial

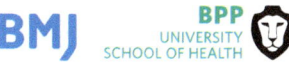

THE BOTTOM LINE

- Inspect the nasal septum after any nasal trauma, no matter how trivial, to assess for a septal haematoma

- Common presenting features include nasal obstruction, pain, rhinorrhea, and fever

- It may be visible as a fluctuant swelling arising from the nasal septum, more commonly (but not always) bilateral

- Refer all patients suspected of having a septal haematoma as an emergency to the ear, nose, and throat department

- Septal haematomas can cause severe cosmetic nasal deformities as well as serious life threatening infective complications

HOW COMMON ARE NASAL SEPTAL HAEMATOMAS?

- The incidence of nasal septal haematomas in primary care is unknown, but it has been reported to occur in 0.8-1.6% of patients with nasal injury who are reviewed by an ear, nose, and throat specialist.[7] Unfortunately, this is likely to be an underestimate because septal haematomas are often undiagnosed, especially in children, until complications occur.[5] [7]

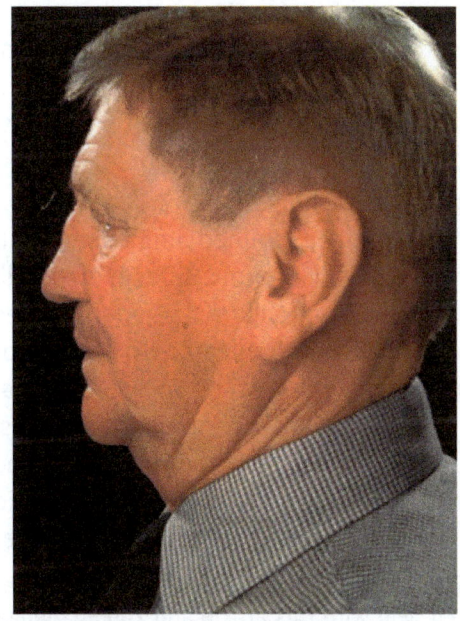

Fig 1 A saddle nose deformity

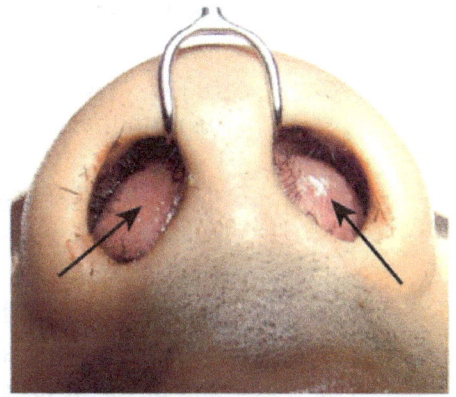

Fig 2 Nasal septal haematoma: what can be seen on simple inspection. With permission from M Kotb (www.drmkotb.com/EN/index.php?page=stu dents&case=&A=2&B=6&C=0)

nasal deformity.[7] Classically, a "saddle" nose deformity (fig 1) is seen, although it may take several years to develop. [13]

Nasal septal abscesses can develop secondary to bacterial colonisation of a septal haematoma and a high proportion of them are thought to be related to previous septal haematomas.[4] [5] Infection of a septal haematoma can occur as early as three days after the formation of a haematoma, and it can intensify subsequent septal necrosis and resorption owing to bacterial proteolytic enzymes.[5] A nasal septal abscess is a serious medical condition. It requires urgent surgical management because it can result in substantial morbidity and mortality. Potentially life threatening complications—such as meningitis, intracranial abscesses, orbital cellulitis, and cavernous sinus thrombosis—can develop because of the venous drainage of the nasal septum.[5] [14] It therefore requires urgent surgical management.

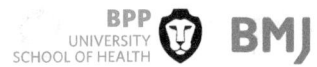

How is a nasal septal haematoma diagnosed?

Clinical features

The presenting symptoms of a nasal septal haematoma are generally non-specific, but the most common presenting symptoms are nasal obstruction (95%), pain (50%), rhinorrhoea (25%), and fever (25%).[12] They can occur after minor trauma, and patients tend to present after nasal injury to either primary care or a minor injuries department.[10] [15] Any patient presenting to primary care with a history of nasal trauma, however minor, should be assessed for the presence of a nasal septal haematoma. All patients suspected of having a septal haematoma should be referred urgently for an ear, nose, and throat assessment.

Investigations

Worsening bilateral nasal obstruction after nasal trauma should immediately raise the suspicion of a septal haematoma. It is diagnosed clinically on direct anterior rhinoscopy (fig 2). A red, fluctuant swelling that obstructs the nasal cavity bilaterally is seen arising from the nasal septum. Unilateral presentation has also been reported. In a primary care setting, an otoscope can be used to visualise the nasal septum. The main differential diagnosis of a nasal septal haematoma is a deviated nasal septum. The two conditions can easily be distinguished by gentle probing with a blunt instrument, such as a cotton bud. A septal haematoma is a boggy swelling, whereas a deviated nasal septum will be firm. Nasal airflow can be assessed easily and simply using a metal tongue depressor or spoon. This is held beneath the anterior nares to look for the presence of two spots of condensation.

How is a nasal septal haematoma managed?

Nasal septal haematomas need to be drained immediately and intravenous antibiotics started to prevent nasal deformity and serious infective complications. This can be done using local anaesthetic in adults, but in children a general anaesthetic is usually required. Necrotic cartilage should be excised and, if infected, the area should be thoroughly irrigated and pus sent for culture and sensitivity testing. To prevent re-accumulation, a corrugated drain can be sutured into the haematoma cavity, drainage holes can be created and nasal packing inserted, or quilting sutures can be fashioned. Nasal packs can be left in place for 2-3 days. The patient will usually require broad spectrum antibiotics for at least one week postoperatively and might benefit from a short course of intravenous treatment.

Acknowledgment: We would like to thank Richard Thomas, senior house officer, Princess of Wales Hospital, Bridgend, for his initial help with this article and Zareena Jedaar, emergency medicine consultant, University Hospital of Wales, Cardiff, for her feedback on the manuscript from a primary care perspective.

Contributors: LNS revised and edited the initial draft of the article, updated it with up to date evidence, and prepared and submitted final article. SEJF had the initial idea for the article and prepared initial draft, performed the initial literature search, and was involved in preparation of final article. PJC provided senior, consultant, supervision by analysing the work and helping to write early drafts and revisions of the manuscripts. LNS and SEJF are the guarantors.

Competing interests: We have read and understood BMJ policy on declaration of interests and declare the following interests: none.

Provenance and peer review: Not commissioned; externally peer reviewed.

Patient consent not required (patient anonymised, dead, or hypothetical). Patient consent obtained for figures.

1   Baring DE, Bowyer DJ, Adamson R. Patient self-assessment of nasal fractures and self referral to an ear, nose, and throat department: a prospective study. *Otolaryngol Head Neck Surg* 2012;146:913-7.
2   Mondin V, Rinaldo A, Ferlito A. Management of nasal bone fractures. *Am J Otolaryngol* 2005;26:181-5.
3   Lee SJ, Liong K, Lee HP. Deformation of nasal septum during nasal trauma. *Laryngoscope* 2010;120:1931-9.
4   Dispenza C, Saraniti C, Dispenza F, Caramanna C, Salzano FA. Management of nasal septal abscess in childhood: our experience. *Int J Pediatr Otorhinolaryngol* 2004;68:1417-21.
5   Alshaikh N, Lo S. Nasal septal abscess in children: from diagnosis to management and prevention. *Int J Pediatr Otorhinolaryngol* 2011;75:737-44.

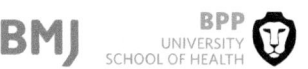

6 Flint PW, Haughey BH, Lund VJ, Niparko JK, Richardson MA, Robbins KT, et al. *Cummings otolaryngology—head and neck surgery* . 5th ed. Mosby, 2010.

7 Alvarez H, Osorio J, De Diego JI, Prim MP, De La Torre C, Gavilan J. Sequelae after nasal septum injuries in children. *Auris Nasus Larynx* 2000;27:339-42.

8 Wright RJ, Murakarmi CS, Ambro BT. Pediatric nasal injuries and management. *Facial Plast Surg* 2011;27:483-90.

9 Chukuezi AB. Nasal septal haematoma in Nigeria. J Laryngol Otol 1992;106:396-8.

10 Olsen KD, Carpenter RJ, Kern EB. Nasal septal injury in children. Diagnosis and management. *Arch Otolaryngol* 1980;106:317-20.

11 Agrawal N, Brayley N. Audit of nasal fracture management in accident and emergency in a district general hospital. *J Eval Clin Pract* 2007;13:295-7.

12 Canty PA, Berkowitz RG. Hematoma and abscess of the nasal septum in children. *Arch Otolaryngol Head Neck Surg* 1996;122:1373-6.

13 Wilson SW, Milward TM. Delayed diagnosis of septal haematoma and consequent nasal deformity. *Injury* 1994;25:685-6.

14 Huang PH, Chiang YC, Yang TH, Chao PZ, Lee FP. Nasal septal abscess. *Otolaryngol Head Neck Surg* 2006;135:335-6.

15 Matsuba HM, Thawley SE. Nasal septal abscess: unusual causes, complications, treatment, and sequelae. *Ann Plast Surg* 1986;16:161-6.

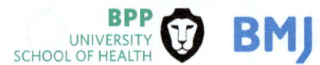

Imported malaria

Merlin L Willcox, general practitioner[1],
Jill Mant, paediatric specialist registrar[2],
Tim O'Dempsey, consultant in tropical medicine[3]

[1]Department of Primary Care Health Sciences, University of Oxford, Oxford OX1 2EP, UK

[2]Department of Paediatrics, Luton Hospital, Luton, UK

[3]Liverpool School of Tropical Medicine, Liverpool, UK

Correspondence to: M L Willcox merlin.willcox@phc.ox.ac.uk

Cite this as: *BMJ* 2013;346:f3214

DOI: 10.1136/bmj.f3214

www.bmj.com/content/346/bmj.f3214

A 19 year old student phoned an official health service telephone helpline with a 10 day history of aching legs, vomiting, diarrhoea, and abdominal pain. She mentioned a recent trip to Uganda but was reassured and told she had "flu." The next day her boyfriend took her to see her doctor, where she mentioned general malaise, tiredness, and occasional nausea; the doctor diagnosed a viral illness and advised her to keep taking paracetamol. Three days later a friend found her dead in bed in her university halls of residence. The coroner recorded death due to cerebral malaria.[1]

What is malaria?

Malaria is an infection caused by protozoa of the genus *Plasmodium*. Five species infect humans (*P falciparum, P vivax, P ovale, P malariae,* and *P knowlesi*). Most of the fatal cases are caused by *P falciparum*.

Why is malaria missed in non-endemic countries?

As illustrated by the case described here, the symptoms of malaria are non-specific and can easily be mistaken for a viral illness such as influenza, unless clinicians think to ask patients whether they have travelled abroad.

A retrospective observational study of 191 deaths due to malaria in the United Kingdom from 1987 to 2006 found that the case fatality was inversely related to incidence, suggesting that cases were more easily missed by clinicians unaccustomed to seeing this disease.[4] A retrospective series of 39 cases of malaria diagnosed in Sheffield from 2000 to 2005 found that eight of these patients had presented to health professionals with symptoms of malaria but were not immediately referred to hospital or for a diagnostic test, suggesting that the diagnosis of malaria had not been considered.[6] A retrospective case review of 211 children admitted to hospital with malaria in east London found that 114 had initially presented to their doctor, but malaria was suspected at the first visit in only 32% of these, and diagnosis was delayed in 53%, by one to 14 days.[7]

Why does this matter?

If untreated, malaria can be rapidly fatal, particularly in non-immune patients. Delay in diagnosis is associated with an increased risk of severe malaria and death.[5] [8] The overall case fatality rate from malaria in the United Kingdom is 0.73%,[4] but for cases with signs of severe malaria (box) this may reach 10-20%.[9] Severe complications and death may occur within 24-48 hours of onset of symptoms.[10] [11] Early diagnosis and appropriate treatment are therefore crucial.

KEY POINTS

- If patients have fever, history of fever, or flu-like symptoms, always ask about travel to a malaria endemic country within the past year
- If malaria is suspected, request urgent thick and thin malaria films (three negative films results on consecutive days are needed to exclude the diagnosis) and a full blood count (thrombocytopaenia is common in acute malaria)
- If there are any signs of severe malaria, admit as an emergency

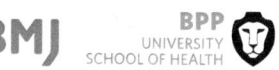

DEFINITION OF SEVERE MALARIA[9]

In patients with *Plasmodium falciparum* asexual parasitaemia and no other obvious cause of symptoms, severe malaria is defined by one or more of the following features:

Clinical features

- Impaired consciousness or coma from which patients cannot be roused
- Prostration—that is, generalised weakness such that that patients cannot sit up unaided
- Failure to feed
- Multiple convulsions—more than two episodes in 24 hours
- Deep breathing, respiratory distress (acidotic breathing)
- Circulatory collapse or shock, systolic blood pressure <70 mm Hg in adults and <50 mm Hg in children
- Clinical jaundice plus evidence of other vital organ dysfunction
- Haemoglobinuria
- Abnormal spontaneous bleeding
- Pulmonary oedema (radiological)

Laboratory findings

Haematology

- Severe normocytic anaemia (haemoglobin level <50 g/L, packed cell volume <15%)
- Hyperparasitaemia (>2% or 100 000/μL in areas of low intensity of transmission; >5% or 250 000/μL in areas of high and stable intensity of transmission)

Biochemistry

- Hypoglycaemia (blood glucose level <2.2 mmol/L or <40 mg/dL)
- Renal impairment (serum creatinine level >265 μmol/L)
- Metabolic acidosis (plasma bicarbonate level <15 mmol/L)
- Hyperlactataemia (lactate >5 mmol/L)

Urine

- Haemoglobinuria

HOW COMMON IS MALARIA?

- Worldwide over 200 million cases of malaria occur annually and 0.5-1 million deaths, 90% of which are among children in Africa[2]
- *Plasmodium falciparum* accounted for about 70% of the 1677 cases notified in the United Kingdom in 2011, whereas 25% of cases were due to *P vivax*[3]
- Of the 191 deaths from malaria in the United Kingdom from 1987 to 2006, 184 were due to *P falciparum*[4]
- About 20% of imported malaria cases are in children[5]

How is malaria diagnosed?

Clinical

Question anyone presenting with a history of fever or flu-like symptoms about travel to malaria endemic countries within the past year. Investigate urgently those returning from a malaria endemic area, regardless of whether they have taken malaria prophylaxis. Intermittent fever may be a feature of malaria, so temperature may be normal at the time of examination. A case series of 482 patients in the United States found that half of adult patients were not febrile when they presented, although most had a history of fever.[12]

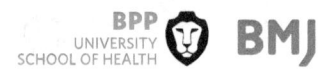

Other common symptoms include vomiting, diarrhoea, headache, and myalgia.[5] [12] Most patients with P falciparum present within six months of returning from abroad, although later presentations may occur. The box shows the features of severe disease.

Investigations

It is preferable to refer all patients with suspected malaria to hospital immediately for further investigation because of the risk of rapid progression of falciparum malaria. However, if the patient is relatively well and it is possible to obtain results rapidly (the same day), it may be reasonable to investigate in a primary care setting. This calls for some clinical judgment. If the risk of malaria is low and the patient is not severely ill, outpatient testing with next day results may be acceptable, but the patient should then be advised to reconsult rapidly if there is any worsening of symptoms.

The clinician should request an urgent full blood count and "malaria thick and thin films" (both on the same EDTA sample). Although microscopy is the standard diagnostic method, low density infection may be missed,[13] particularly if microscopists are inexperienced or if patients have taken an antimalarial or an antibiotic with antimalarial activity. Therefore, if the first slide gives a negative result, films should be repeated after 12-24 hours, and again after another 24 hours. The likelihood of malaria is low if experienced microscopists find three consecutive negative blood film results.[14]

In the United Kingdom some haematology laboratories may also be able to perform a rapid diagnostic test. These tests are based on detection of parasite antigens or enzymes; a recent Cochrane review found that the sensitivity and specificity of the most common rapid diagnostic tests were both 95%, compared with microscopy.[15] Rapid diagnostic tests are useful in increasing speed of diagnosis, even in non-endemic countries[16] and, if available, can be used as an adjunct to microscopy, although they cannot replace it. All positive malaria test results should be telephoned immediately to the requesting doctor and communicated by the doctor to the patient.[14]

Thrombocytopenia is common in acute malaria, and, if otherwise unexplained, may be an important clue even if the blood film has been reported as negative. A prospective study looking at returning travellers with fever found that leucocyte counts $<10\times10^9$/L, platelet counts $<150\times10^9$/L, and haemoglobin levels <120 g/L were all associated with an increased probability of malaria. Thrombocytopenia was the best predictor, with a positive likelihood ratio of 11.[17]

How is malaria managed?

Seek expert advice on treatment, particularly if there are signs of complications. In the primary care setting, if there are any signs of severe malaria, refer the patient to hospital as an emergency and treat any complications (for example, shock, hypoglycaemia, convulsions) while awaiting transfer.

Most patients with falciparum malaria need admission to hospital, although recent evidence has suggested that a small selected group with uncomplicated falciparum malaria can be treated safely as outpatients.[18] [19] Those with uncomplicated non-falciparum infections can usually be managed as outpatients provided they are able to take oral drugs. Mixed infections can occur and P falciparum may be missed or misdiagnosed. Therefore it is sensible to have a low threshold for admission and to advise all those treated as outpatients to seek further medical attention urgently if they deteriorate. It is also advisable to review all patients with malaria 1-2 weeks after completion of treatment.[18] [19]

Because of the risk of increasing drug resistance, the World Health Organization now recommends that uncomplicated P falciparum malaria should be treated with artemisinin combination therapies.[9] Recent studies have proved that intravenous artesunate is more effective than quinine for the treatment of severe malaria,[20] [21] but UK guidelines still recommend quinine because artesunate is unlicensed in the European Union.[14] These guidelines are, however, currently under review. Chloroquine is usually effective for non-falciparum malarias; however, chloroquine resistant *P vivax* is increasingly prevalent in some areas (for example, Indonesia, Peru, and Oceania).[9] In addition, patients with *P vivax* or *P ovale* infections should have their glucose 6 phosphate dehydrogenase (G6PD) status checked and, unless significantly G6PD deficient, should also be treated with an appropriate course of primaquine to reduce the likelihood of relapses.[22]

UK guidelines for malaria treatment[14] and a useful management algorithm are available at www.hpa.org.uk/Topics/InfectiousDiseases/InfectionsAZ/Malaria/Guidelines/mala20guidelinesTreatment/.

Contributors: MW wrote the first draft of the article, which was revised by the coauthors. All authors read and approved the final manuscript. MW is guarantor of the paper.

Competing interests: All authors have completed the ICMJE uniform disclosure form at http://www.icmje.org/coi_disclosure.pdf (available on request from the corresponding author) and declare: no support from any organisation for the submitted work; no financial relationships with any organisations that might have an interest in the submitted work in the previous three years, no other relationships or activities that could appear to have influenced the submitted work.

Provenance and peer review: Not commissioned; externally peer reviewed.

Patient consent not required (patient anonymised, dead, or hypothetical).

1 Anon. Student died of Malaria after being diagnosed with flu. Secondary student died of malaria after being diagnosed with flu. *Mail Online* 2007 Jan 10. www.dailymail.co.uk/news/article-427932/Student-died-Malaria-diagnosed-flu.html#.
2 World Health Organization. World malaria report 2011. WHO, 2011.
3 Health Protection Agency. Imported malaria cases and deaths, United Kingdom: 1992-2011. Secondary imported malaria cases and deaths, United Kingdom: 1992-2011. 2012. www.hpa.org.uk/Topics/InfectiousDiseases/InfectionsAZ/Malaria/EpidemiologicalData/malaEpi10CasesandDeaths/.
4 Checkley AM, Smith A, Smith V, Blaze M, Bradley D, Chiodini PL, et al. Risk factors for mortality from imported falciparum malaria in the United Kingdom over 20 years: an observational study. *BMJ* 2012;344:bmj.e2116.
5 Ladhani S, Aibara RJ, Riordan FA, Shingadia D. Imported malaria in children: a review of clinical studies. *Lancet Infect Dis* 2007;7:349-57.
6 Green ST, Jary HR, Darton TC. Missed opportunities to diagnose Plasmodium falciparum malaria: results of a regional service evaluation. *J Infect* 2009;58:172-3.
7 Ladhani S, El Bashir H, Patel VS, Shingadia D. Childhood malaria in East London. *Pediatr Infect Dis J* 2003;22:814-9.
8 Dubos F, Dauriac A, El Mansouf L, Courouble C, Aurel M, Martinot A. Imported malaria in children: incidence and risk factors for severity. *Diagn Microbiol Infect Dis* 2010;66:169-74.
9 World Health Organization. Guidelines for the treatment of malaria. 2 edn. WHO, 2010.
10 Centers for Disease Control and Prevention. Domestic refugee health guidelines: malaria. secondary domestic refugee health guidelines: malaria. 2012. www.cdc.gov/immigrantrefugeehealth/guidelines/domestic/malaria-guidelines-domestic.html.
11 Newman RD, Parise ME, Barber AM, Steketee RW. Malaria-related deaths among U.S. travelers, 1963-2001. *Ann Intern Med* 2004;141:547-55.
12 Svenson JE, MacLean JD, Gyorkos TW, Keystone J. Imported malaria. Clinical presentation and examination of symptomatic travelers. *Arch Intern Med* 1995;155:861-8.
13 Batwala V, Magnussen P, Nuwaha F. Are rapid diagnostic tests more accurate in diagnosis of plasmodium falciparum malaria compared to microscopy at rural health centres? *Malar J* 2010;9:349.
14 Lalloo DG, Shingadia D, Pasvol G, Chiodini PL, Whitty CJ, Beeching NJ, et al. UK malaria treatment guidelines. *J Infect* 2007;54:111-21.
15 Abba K, Deeks JJ, Olliaro P, Naing CM, Jackson SM, Takwoingi Y, et al. Rapid diagnostic tests for diagnosing uncomplicated P. falciparum malaria in endemic countries. *Cochrane Database Syst Rev* 2011;(7):CD008122.
16 Rossi I, D'Acremont V, Prod'Hom G, Genton B. Safety of falciparum malaria diagnostic strategy based on rapid diagnostic tests in returning travellers and migrants: a retrospective study. *Malar J* 2012;11:377.
17 D'Acremont V, Landry P, Mueller I, Pecoud A, Genton B. Clinical and laboratory predictors of imported malaria in an outpatient setting: an aid to medical decision making in returning travelers with fever. *Am J Trop Med Hyg* 2002;66:481-6.
18 Bottieau E, Clerinx J, Colebunders R, Van den Enden E, Wouters R, Demey H, et al. Selective ambulatory management of imported falciparum malaria: a 5-year prospective study. *Eur J Clin Microbiol Infect Dis* 2007;26:181-8.
19 Kiang KM, Bryant PA, Shingadia D, Ladhani S, Steer AC, Burgner D. The treatment of imported malaria in children: an update. *Arch Dis Child Educ Pract Ed* 2013;98:7-15.
20 Dondorp A, Nosten F, Stepniewska K, Day N, White N, South East Asian Quinine Artesunate Malaria Trial (SEAQUAMAT) group. Artesunate versus quinine for treatment of severe falciparum malaria: a randomised trial. *Lancet* 2005;366:717-25.

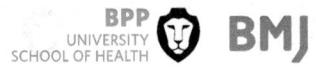

21 Dondorp AM, Fanello CI, Hendriksen ICE, Gomes E, Seni A, Chhaganlal KD, et al. Artesunate versus quinine in the treatment of severe falciparum malaria in African children (AQUAMAT): an open-label, randomised trial. *Lancet* 2010;376:1647-57.

22 British Medical Association, Royal Pharmaceutical Society of Great Britain. British national formulary. London: BMA, RPS, 2013:422, 428. (No 65.)

Related links

bmj.com/archive
Previous articles in this series

- Spontaneous oesophageal rupture (2013;346:f3095)
- Pelvic inflammatory disease (2013;346:f3189)
- Colorectal cancer (2013;346:f3172)
- Acute leg ischaemia (2013;346:f2681)
- Delirium in older adults (2013;346:f2031)

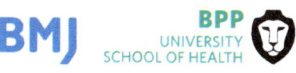

Joint hypermobility syndrome

Juliette Ross, GP principal[1],

Rodney Grahame, consultant rheumatologist[2], honorary professor[3], affiliate professor of pathology[4]

[1]Wembley Park Drive Medical Centre, Wembley, UK

[2]Hypermobility Clinic, University College Hospital, London NW1 2PQ, UK

[3]Department of Medicine, University College London, London

[4]School of Medicine, University of Washington, Seattle, WA, USA

Correspondence to: R Grahame rodney. grahame@uclh.nhs.uk

Cite this as: BMJ 2011;342:c7167

DOI: 10.1136/bmj.c7167

www.bmj.com/content/342/bmj.c7167

Joint hypermobility syndrome (JHS), previously known as benign joint hypermobility syndrome (BJHS), is a heritable disorder of connective tissue that comprises symptomatic hypermobility predisposing to arthralgia, soft tissue injury, and joint instability.[1] It is indistinguishable from the hypermobility type of Ehlers-Danlos syndrome.[2] Complications may include autonomic dysfunction, proprioceptive impairment, premature osteoarthritis, intestinal dysmotility, and laxity in other tissues causing hernias or uterine or rectal prolapse. Symptoms are often minimal or mild, but 168 out of 700 patients with joint hypermobility syndrome (24%) attending the UCH Hypermobility Clinic already had an established chronic pain syndrome at the time of their first outpatient attendance. These patients were experiencing serious pain, disability, and impairment of the quality of life, some patients becoming chairbound or even bedbound.[3]

Why is it missed?

In a recent survey among members of the Hypermobility Syndrome Association (a patient self help group), largely due to missed diagnosis, 52% of 251 patients waited over 10 years from the onset of symptoms to get a correct diagnosis.[11]

Doctors may be unaware of the prevalence of the condition, its effect on quality of life, or its multisystemic nature (box 2) and may not routinely look for hypermobility in the clinical examination, especially as the condition rarely forms part of the curriculum in medical schools or in postgraduate training programmes for general practitioners, specialists, or physiotherapists or occupational therapists.[12] The erroneous view that hypermobility is a variant of normality, rather than part of an inherited connective tissue disorder, is also still widely held. In a survey of 319 UK consultant rheumatologists, only 9% of respondents believed that joint hypermobility syndrome and the hypermobility type of Ehlers-Danlos syndrome were the same condition. Furthermore, 46% of respondents were sceptical about a serious impact on people's lives and 72% about a serious contribution to the overall burden of rheumatic disease.[13]

Why does this matter?

If joint hypermobility syndrome is missed, the following problems may arise:

- Inappropriate and potentially harmful labelling or treatments may be applied on the basis of an erroneous diagnosis such as rheumatoid arthritis, hypochondriasis, or somatisation.

- Over zealous physical manipulation may cause avoidable damage, such as (a) precipitating subluxation or dislocation of intervertebral or peripheral joints, (b) inflicting rupture on ligaments, joint capsules, muscles, or tendons, or (c) precipitating pathological fractures in fragile bone. Exercise therapy may be either excessively forceful or ineffectual.[14]

- Anecdotal evidence exists that orthopaedic operations may be done without the surgeon knowing that the patient has an underlying connective tissue disorder, and this may lead to poorer outcomes.

- Chronic pain may sometimes lead to a potentially reversible downward spiral of immobility, deconditioning, dependency, and despair.[5] Out of 700 patients with joint hypermobility syndrome (24%) attending the UCH Hypermobility Clinic, 168 were experiencing serious pain, disability, and impairment of the quality of life, some patients becoming chairbound or even bedbound.[3]

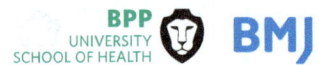

> ### BOX 1 NINE-POINT BEIGHTON SCORE FOR JOINT HYPERMOBILITY SYNDROME[4]
>
> One point is gained for each side of the body for the first four manoeuvres listed below, such that the hypermobility score is a maximum of 9 if all are positive.
>
> - Passive dorsiflexion of the fifth metacarpophalangeal joint to .90° (1 point for left; 1 point for right) (A)
>
> - Opposition of the thumb to the volar aspect of the ipsilateral forearm (1 point for left; 1 point for right) (fig 1B)
>
> - Hyperextension of the elbow to .10° (1 point for left; 1 point for right) (fig 1C)
>
> - Hyperextension of the knee to .10° (1 point for left; 1 point for right) (fig 1D)
>
> - Placing of hands flat on the floor without bending the knees (1 point) (fig 1E)

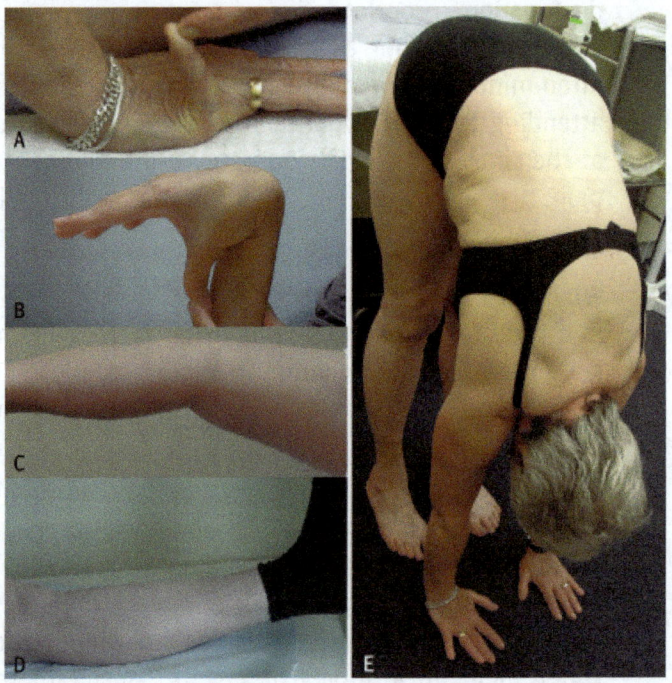

Fig 1 Patients illustrate the application of the nine point Beighton hypermobility score.[5] Adapted with permission from Springer Science+Business Media

How is it diagnosed?

Diagnosis is entirely clinical as currently no biological or imaging markers are available. The musculoskeletal symptoms mainly derive from a vulnerability to injury resulting from fragile collagenous tissues (tendon, ligament, muscle, bone, cartilage, and skin). In patients with arthralgia or post-injury musculoskeletal pain, screening blood tests and/or appropriate imaging are needed to exclude conditions such as inflammatory arthritis and fractures. Box 3 lists important common clues to joint hypermobility syndrome. The Beighton score (box 1) identifies joint hypermobility but is too insensitive an instrument for diagnosing joint hypermobility syndrome and is not intended for this purpose. Diagnosis requires the application of the 1998 Brighton criteria into which the Beighton score has been incorporated (box 2).[6] The reproducibility and reliability of the Beighton score and the Brighton criteria have recently been scrutinised,[15 16 17] and an international panel is currently reviewing the Brighton criteria.[17]

How is it managed?

The key players are the family doctor and a suitably trained physiotherapist.

Doctor's role

- To establish an accurate diagnosis of joint hypermobility syndrome while being alert to the possibility of one of the rarer and more serious heritable disorders of connective tissue, such as Marfan's syndrome, or other forms of Ehlers-Danlos syndrome, such as vascular,

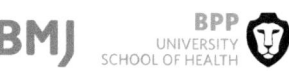

> **BOX 2 1998 BRIGHTON CRITERIA FOR CLASSIFICATION OF JOINT HYPERMOBILITY SYNDROME*[6]**
>
> Joint hypermobility syndrome is diagnosed in the presence of two major criteria; one major criterion plus two minor criteria; or four minor criteria. Two minor criteria will suffice where there is an unequivocally affected first degree relative.
>
> The syndrome is excluded by the presence of Marfan's or Ehlers-Danlos syndromes (other than the hypermobility type of Ehlers-Danlos syndrome) as defined by the Ghent 1996[7] and Villefranche 1998[8] criteria respectively.
>
> **Major criteria**
> - Beighton score of ≥4 (either currently or previously)
> - Arthralgia for longer than three months in four or more joints
>
> **Minor criteria**
> - Beighton score of 1, 2, or 3 (0, 1, 2, or 3 if aged ›50 years)
> - Arthralgia in one to three joints or back pain or spondylosis, spondylolysis and/or spondylolisthesis
> - Dislocation in more than one joint or in one joint on more than one occasion
> - Three or more soft tissue lesions (eg, epicondylitis, tenosynovitis, bursitis)
> - Marfanoid habitus (tall, slim, ratio of span to height greater than 1.03 and/or ratio of upper segment to lower segment less than 0.89, arachnodactyly)
> - Abnormal skin: striae, hyperextensibility, thin skin, papyraceous scarring
> - Eye signs: drooping eyelids, myopia, or antimongoloid slant
> - Varicose veins, hernia, or uterine or rectal prolapse
>
> *Although originally designed for use as a research tool in defining a cohort of patients for recruitment into clinical studies, in practice the criteria have proved to be a useful diagnostic aid in the clinical setting.*

or classical. A positive family history of sudden early death from aortic aneurysmal dissection and/or rupture should suggest the possibility of Marfan's syndrome, and a history of major spontaneous arterial rupture or uterine rupture in childbirth should raise suspicions of the vascular type of Ehlers-Danlos syndrome.

- To make a detailed assessment of the effects of the disorder on musculoskeletal function, systemic involvement (such as dysautonomia, gastrointestinal dysmotility), declining mobility, and quality of life.

Physiotherapist's role:
- To adapt physiotherapy principles to the needs of patients with lax and fragile tissues. This involves:
- Core and joint stabilising and proprioception enhancing exercises
- General fitness training to offset or reverse the tendency for the body to lose condition
- The use of mobilising techniques to restore natural hypermobility to joints or spinal segments where these have been lost as a result of deconditioning and kinesiophobia.[28]

A before and after comparison study in 18 patients from Glasgow with joint hypermobility syndrome has shown that a home based programme of specific exercises may improve proprioception, symptoms, and quality of life.[29]

For patients with chronic pain for which analgesics are largely ineffective, a pain management programme based on cognitive behavioural techniques and delivered by a specially trained pain psychologist may reduce pain catastrophising, anxiety, and interference of pain with daily life.[30]

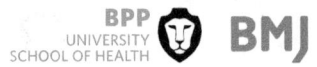

BOX 3 COMMON CLUES SUGGESTING JOINT HYPERMOBILITY SYNDROME (BASED ON OBSERVATIONS, EXPERT OPINION, AND CASE SERIES)

In children and adolescents
- Coincidental congenital dislocation of the hip[18]
- Late walking, with bottom shuffling instead of crawling[19]
- Recurrent ankle sprains[20]
- Poor ball catching and handwriting skills[21]
- Tiring easily compared with peers
- So called growing pains or chronic widespread pain[21]
- Joint dislocations[22]

In adults
- Non-inflammatory joint or spinal pain[23]
- Joint dislocations[22]
- Multiple soft tissue (including sporting) injuries[24]
- Increase in pain or progressive intensification of pain that is largely unresponsive to analgesics[5]
- Progressive loss of mobility owing to pain or kinesiophobia (pain avoidance through movement avoidance)[5]
- Premature osteoarthritis[25]
- Autonomic dysfunction, such as orthostatic intolerance (dizziness or faintness) or postural tachycardia syndrome (in this form of dysautonomia, in 60° upright tilt the blood pressure remains constant while the pulse rate rises by a minimum of 30 beats/min)
- Functional gastrointestinal disorders (sluggish bowel, bloating, rectal evacuatory dysfunction)[26]
- Laxity in other supporting tissues—for example, hernias, varicose veins, or uterine or rectal prolapse[27]

CASE SCENARIO

A 30 year old project manager, who is new to your general practice, presents with right anterior knee pain after slipping and landing on his knee three months ago. Imaging shows no abnormality, but he describes a long history of recurrent shoulder subluxation, and many soft tissue problems and joint pains, often after similarly trivial trauma, and he states that imaging and blood tests "for arthritis" have always been normal. You note that he has no signs of inflammation but that he is hypermobile according to the Beighton score (see box 1), and looking up the Brighton criteria, which includes and extends the older Beighton score (see box 2), you mention he fulfils the criteria for joint hypermobility syndrome, and he expresses relief there is an explanation for his symptoms.

HOW COMMON IS IT?

Joint hypermobility is very common, occurring in 10-20% of populations of Western countries, and higher still in those in Indian, Chinese, and Middle Eastern groups. It is important to distinguish between joint hypermobility and joint hypermobility syndrome. People who are hypermobile without symptoms are merely people with hypermobility. Those with symptoms attributable to their hypermobility may have joint hypermobility syndrome if they conform to the Brighton criteria. The true prevalence of the syndrome is unknown. In surveys in London and in Santiago, Chile, routine searches in consecutive patients referred to general rheumatology clinics have found prevalences of joint hypermobility syndrome (as defined by the Brighton criteria) as high as 45%; the syndrome is higher in females and non-white people.[9] [10] Therefore many patients presenting to their doctors with common, everyday, noninflammatory, painful, musculoskeletal conditions probably have unrecognised joint hypermobility syndrome.

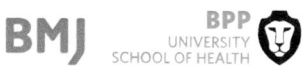

For patients with foot or hand problems, refer to a podiatrist for a mechanical foot assessment and tailor made orthotics[31] or to an occupational therapist for help with writing and other work related hand problems.

Competing interests: Both authors have completed the Unified Competing Interest form at www.icmje.org/coi_disclosure.pdf (available on request from the corresponding author) and declare: no support from any organisation for the submitted work; no financial relationships with any organisations that might have an interest in the submitted work in the previous three years; no other relationships or activities that could appear to have influenced the submitted work.

Provenance and peer review: Commissioned; externally peer reviewed.

Patient consent not required (patient anonymised, dead, or hypothetical).

1   Hakim A, Grahame R. Joint hypermobility. *Best Pract Res Clin Rheumatol* 2003;17:989-1004.
2   Tinkle BT, Bird H, Grahame R, Lavallee M, Levy HP, Sillence D. The lack of clinical distinction between the hypermobility type of Ehlers-Danlos syndrome and the joint hypermobility syndrome (a.k.a. hypermobility syndrome). *Am J Med Genet A* 2009;149A:2368-70.
3   Grahame R. What is the joint hypermobility syndrome? JHS from the cradle to the grave. In: Hakim A, Keer R, Grahame R, eds. Hypermobility, fibromyalgia and chronic pain. Elsevier, 2010.
4   Beighton P, Solomon L, Soskolne CL. Articular mobility in an African population. *Ann Rheum Dis* 1973;32:413-8.
5   Grahame R. Joint hypermobility syndrome pain. *Curr Pain Headache Rep* 2009;13:427-33.
6   Grahame R, Bird HA, Child A. The revised (Brighton 1998) criteria for the diagnosis of benign joint hypermobility syndrome (BJHS). *J Rheumatol* 2000;27:1777-9.
7   De Paepe, Devereux RB, Dietz HC, Hennekam RC, Pyeritz RE. Revised diagnostic criteria for the Marfan syndrome. *Am J Med Genet* 1996;62:417-26.
8   Beighton P, De Paepe A, Steinmann B, Tsipouras P, Wenstrup RJ. Ehlers-Danlos syndromes: revised nosology, Villefranche, 1997. Ehlers-Danlos National Foundation (USA) and Ehlers-Danlos Support Group (UK). *Am J Med Genet* 1998;77:31-7.
9   Grahame R, Hakim AJ. Joint hypermobility syndrome is highly prevalent in general rheumatology clinics, its occurrence and clinical presentation being gender, age and race-related. *Ann Rheum Dis* 2006;65(suppl 2):263.
10 Bravo JF, Wolff C. Clinical study of hereditary disorders of connective tissues in a Chilean population: joint hypermobility syndrome and vascular Ehlers-Danlos syndrome. *Arthritis Rheum* 2006;54:515-23.
11 Hypermobility Syndrome Association, UK. www.hypermobility.org/forum/viewtopic.php?f=3&t=4468.
12 Coady D, Walker D, Kay L. Regional examination of the musculoskeletal system (REMS): a core set of clinical skills for medical students. *Rheumatology (Oxford)* 2004;43:633-9.
13 Grahame R, Bird H. British consultant rheumatologists' perceptions about the hypermobility syndrome: a national survey. *Rheumatology (Oxford)* 2001;40:559-62.
14 Maillard S, Payne J. Physiotherapy and occupational therapy in the hypermobile child. In: Hakim A, Keer R, Grahame R, ed. Hypermobility, fibromyalgia and chronic pain. Elsevier, 2010.
15 Remvig L, Jensen DV, Ward RC. Are diagnostic criteria for general joint hypermobility and benign joint hypermobility syndrome based on reproducible and valid tests? A review of the literature. *J Rheumatol* 2007;34:798-803.
16 Juul-Kristensen B, Rogind H, Jensen DV, Remvig L. Inter-examiner reproducibility of tests and criteria for generalized joint hypermobility and benign joint hypermobility syndrome. *Rheumatology (Oxford)* 2007;46:1835-41.
17 Remvig L, Jensen DV, Ward RC. Epidemiology of general joint hypermobility and basis for the proposed criteria for benign joint hypermobility syndrome: review of the literature. *J Rheumatol* 2007;34:804-9.
18 Wynne-Davies R. Familial joint laxity. *Proc R Soc Med* 1971;64:689-90.
19 Davidovitch M, Tirosh E, Tal Y. The relationship between joint hypermobility and neurodevelopmental attributes in elementary school children. *J Child Neurol* 1994;9:417-9.
20 Diaz MA, Estevez BC, Sanchez-Guijo P. Joint hyperlaxity and musculoligamentous lesions: study of a population of homogenous age, sex and physical exertion. *Br J Rheumatol* 1993;32:120-2.
21 Adib N, Davies K, Grahame R, Woo P, Murray KJ. Joint hypermobility syndrome in childhood. A not so benign multisystem disorder? *Rheumatology (Oxford)* 2005;44:744-50.
22 Runow A. The dislocating patella. Etiology and prognosis in relation to generalized joint laxity and anatomy of the patellar articulation. *Acta Orthop Scand Suppl* 1983;201:1-53.
23 Grahame R, Hakim AJ. Joint hypermobility syndrome is highly prevalent in general rheumatology clinics, its occurrence and clinical presentation being gender, age and race-related. *Ann Rheum Dis* 2006;65(suppl 2):263.
24 Hudson N, Starr MR, Esdaile JM, Fitzcharles MA. Diagnostic associations with hypermobility in rheumatology patients. *Br J Rheumatol* 1995;34:1157-61.
25 Bridges AJ, Smith E, Reid J. Joint hypermobility in adults referred to rheumatology clinics. *Ann Rheum Dis* 1992;51:793-6.

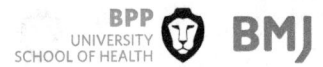

26 Zarate N, Farmer AD, Grahame R, Mohammed S, Knowles CH, Scott SM, et al. Unexplained gastrointestinal symptoms and joint hypermobility: is connective tissue the missing link? *Neurogastroenterol Motil* 2010;22:252-62.

27 Norton PA, Baker JE, Sharp HC, Warenski JC. Genitourinary prolapse and joint hypermobility in women. *Obstet Gynecol* 1995;85:225-8.

28 Simmonds JV, Keer RJ. Hypermobility and the hypermobility syndrome. *Man Ther* 2007;12:298-309.

29 Ferrell WR, Tennant N, Sturrock RD, Ashton L, Creed G, Brydson G, et al. Amelioration of symptoms by enhancement of proprioception in patients with joint hypermobility syndrome. *Arthritis Rheum* 2004;50:3323-8.

30 Daniel HC. Pain management and cognitive behavioural therapy. In: Hakim A, Keer R, Grahame R, ed. Hypermobility, fibromyalgia and chronic pain. Elsevier, 2010.

31 McCulloch R, Redmond A. The hypermobile foot. In: Hakim A, Keer R, Grahame R, ed. Hypermobility, fibromyalgia and chronic pain. Elsevier, 2010.

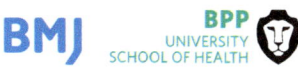

Cholesteatoma

Mahmood F Bhutta, clinical research fellow[1], visiting scientist[2],

Ian G Williamson, clinical senior lecturer[3],

Holger H Sudhoff, professor of otolaryngology/head and neck surgery[4]

[1]Nuffield Department of Surgical Sciences (University of Oxford), John Radcliffe Hospital, Oxford OX3 9DU, UK

[2]MRC Harwell, Harwell Science and Innovation Campus, UK

[3]School of Medicine, University of Southampton, Southampton, UK

[4]Bielefeld Academic Teaching Hospital, Münster University, D-33604 Bielefeld, Germany

Correspondence to: M F Bhutta m.bhutta@doctors.org.uk

Cite this as: BMJ 2011;342:d1088

DOI: 10.1136/bmj.d1088

www.bmj.com/content/342/bmj.d1088

A cholesteatoma is a lesion of the ear, formed of a mass of stratified keratinising squamous epithelium (fig 1).[1] Aetiology is debated,[2] but cholesteatoma probably arises from the lateral epithelium of the tympanic membrane, and then grows as a self perpetuating mass into the middle ear. This may activate local osteoclasts,[3] possibly as a result of infection of dead epithelium at the centre of the lesion, with potentially serious consequences from local tissue destruction.

Why is cholesteatoma missed?

The onset of disease may be insidious with intermittent or mild symptoms. Typically cholesteatoma presents with intermittent unilateral otorrhoea (ear discharge) and a progressive hearing loss,[6] which may mimic and be misdiagnosed as recurrent or chronic otitis externa or otitis media. Successful negligence claims have been filed in the United Kingdom (http://boyesturnerclaims.com/case-study.html?id=85) and the United States (www.upton-hatfield.com/news/verdicts.html) for complications resulting from a missed diagnosis in primary care, although no published data are available on frequency of misdiagnosis.

Why does it matter?

A cholesteatoma is a self perpetuating mass, which if untreated, can cause extensive local tissue destruction. At presentation the ossicles are often eroded, contributing to conductive hearing loss.[7] Rarely cholesteatoma may erode into the inner ear causing sensorineural hearing loss or vertigo, or lead to facial palsy from damage to the facial nerve as it traverses the middle ear.[8] Cholesteatoma can also lead to spread of infection through the tegmen (roof) of the middle ear causing meningitis or intracranial abscess (fig 2), a risk estimated to be 1 in 10 000 a year of untreated disease.[9]

How is cholesteatoma diagnosed?

Clinical features

Symptoms of cholesteatoma—such as persistent hearing loss (present in 83% of 23 ears in a case series), otorrhoea (56%), otalgia (39%), vertigo, or tinnitus—are non-specific,[6] and so the diagnosis rests on the appearance on otoscopic examination. Cholesteatoma is classically described as "wax in the attic": a yellow or white crust visible in the upper part (pars flaccida or "attic") of the tympanic membrane, often surrounded by pus, and with a perforation of the adjacent tympanic membrane and erosion of the surrounding bone (fig 1). In advanced cases, bony erosion may be severe and normal anatomy difficult to recognise. Whereas most cholesteatomas arise in the attic, they can also arise in the lower part (pars tensa) of the tympanic membrane.[7]

KEY POINTS

- Cholesteatoma is a locally destructive lesion of the middle ear, in the form of a cyst of keratinous epithelium
- Cholesteatoma can occasionally lead to serious consequences, including facial palsy, meningitis, or brain abscess
- It should be suspected in any case of persistent or recurrent ear discharge
- The key to diagnosis is a characteristic appearance on otoscopy

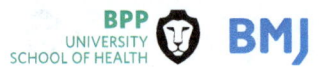

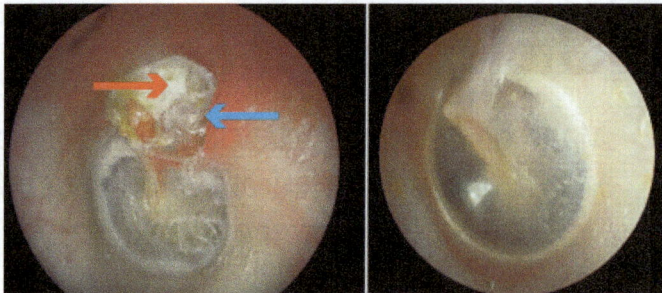

Fig 1 Left: Cholesteatoma (red arrow) arising in the upper part (pars flaccida or "attic") of left tympanic membrane. Note erosion of surrounding bone (blue arrow). Right: Normal tympanic membrane (left ear) for comparison

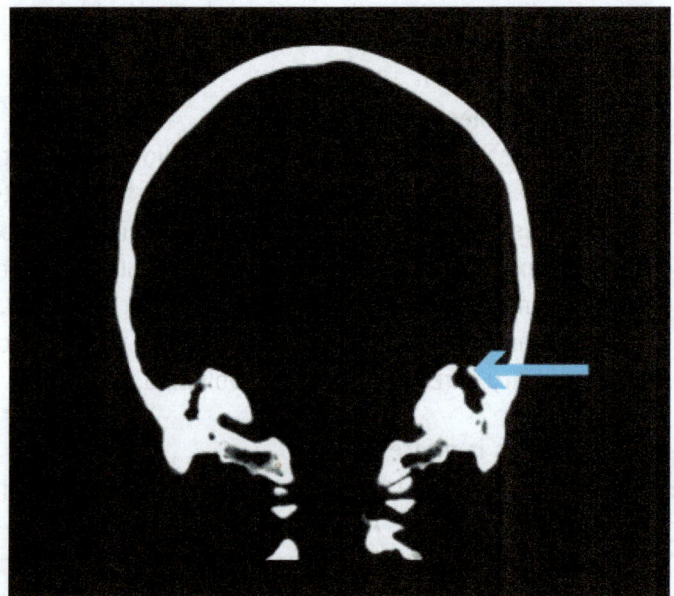

Fig 2 Sagittal computed tomogram through the temporal bones of a patient with longstanding left cholesteatoma. The bony tegmen (roof) of the left middle ear has eroded (arrow), leading to an abscess in the temporal lobe

---

HOW COMMON IS CHOLESTEATOMA?

- The estimated incidence of cholesteatoma in northern Europe is 9.2 per 100000 population a year[4]

- Therefore a general practitioner with a practice size of 2500 patients would be expected to see on average one new case every four to five years

- The peak incidence is in the age range 5-15 years,[5] but cholesteatoma can arise in any age group

- Seven per cent of people diagnosed will subsequently develop cholesteatoma in the contralateral ear[5]

- The incidence is reportedly higher in white than non-white populations.

CASE SCENARIO

A 24 year old man presented to his general practitioner several times over a year with an intermittently discharging left ear and associated hearing loss. Visualisation of the tympanic membrane was not possible owing to otorrhoea and oedema in the external auditory canal. He was treated for presumed otitis externa with repeated courses of topical antibiotic drops, but as improvement was only temporary he was referred to a specialist. An otolaryngologist cleared the external auditory canal of debris ("aural toilet") and discovered a cholesteatoma arising from the left tympanic membrane; this was successfully treated by surgical excision.

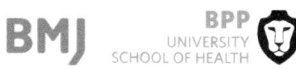

In primary care, cholesteatoma should be suspected in an ear with recurrent or persistent otorrhoea that fails to settle fully with treatment. In general practice such symptoms are more often the result of recurrent otitis externa or recurrent otitis media,[10] but only a full visualisation of the tympanic membrane allows cholesteatoma to be excluded. In all new cases of facial palsy otoscopy should be used to exclude cholesteatoma as a cause.[11]

Visualisation, however, may be difficult. When a cholesteatoma is temporarily or permanently active, the external auditory canal may become filled with purulent discharge and be oedematous, and if facilities are not available for aural toilet, obtaining an adequate view of the tympanic membrane may be impossible. Chronic inflammation may also cause the formation of a macroscopic polyp of granulation tissue,[12] which again can obstruct the view. In paediatric cases the child may not permit examination. In difficult cases it is worth treating the ear for a presumed infection and bringing the patient back for re-examination of the ear once infection has settled. When visualisation is still difficult and symptoms continue, refer the patient to an otolaryngologist for aural toilet or application of topical steroid creams to granulation tissue (possibly under general anaesthesia for a child); this will allow the tympanic membrane to be seen and the presence or absence of cholesteatoma verified.

Investigations

High resolution computed tomography can help to define the likely extent of a cholesteatoma, and it may show bony erosion, which makes the diagnosis more likely.[13] It may also show complications from more advanced disease. Diffusion weighted magnetic resonance imaging has also been used to show cholesteatoma.[14] However, no imaging is sufficiently sensitive or specific for cholesteatoma,[15] and the cornerstone of diagnosis remains clinical, based on the appearance on otoscopy.

An audiogram is needed to define the degree and type of hearing loss. Typically a conductive hearing loss is found, as a result of the cholesteatoma mass itself or erosion of ossicles, but an additional sensorineural hearing loss may be present if the cochlea has also sustained damage.

How is it managed?

When cholesteatoma is diagnosed or suspected, "semi-urgent" referral (for the patient to be seen by a specialist within a few weeks) is appropriate. However, if facial palsy is also present, refer immediately, because if the palsy is caused by the cholesteatoma, delayed treatment is associated with a worse prognosis.[16] [17] [18] The presence of pain or other neurological symptoms or signs should also prompt urgent referral as these may portend intracranial complications.

Surgical excision is the only known cure for cholesteatoma, and the choice of operation depends on the extent of the lesion. Local excision may be sufficient for early cholesteatoma, but more extensive disease requires exploration of the mastoid air cells with a mastoidectomy. This sometimes means that the mastoid air cells are "externalised" by surgical excision of the posterior external auditory canal, to form a mastoid cavity. The risk of residual disease after surgery varies (5% to 30%) with the procedure and extent of the disease, and patients require follow-up and sometimes repeat exploratory surgery.

In some older patients and in patients with concurrent morbidity, conservative management of cholesteatoma may be an option, but as highlighted above, this carries a small but continuing risk of serious complications from this disease.

Thanks to David Pothier for providing the images in figure 1.

Contributors: MFB conceptualised the article and researched and wrote the first draft. IGW and HHS made important revisions.

Funding: No additional funding.

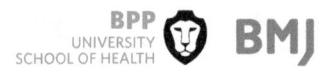

Competing interests: All authors have completed the Unified Competing Interest form at www. icmje.org/coi_disclosure.pdf (available on request from the corresponding author) and declare: no support from any company for the submitted work; IGW has previously received an honorarium from GlaxoSmithKline for a symposium on prescribing in otitis media; and no non-financial interests that may be relevant to the submitted work.

Provenance and peer review: Not commissioned; externally peer reviewed.

Patient consent not required (patient anonymised, dead, or hypothetical).

1   Browning GG, Merchant SM, Kelly G, Swan IRC, Canter R, McKerrow WS. Chronic otitis media. In: Gleeson MJ, ed. *Scott-Brown's otorhinolaryngology, head and neck surgery* . 7th ed. Hodder Arnold, 2008:3395-445.

2   Olszewska E, Wagner M, Bernal-Sprekelsen M, Ebmeyer J, Dazert S, Hildmann H, et al. Etiopathogenesis of cholesteatoma. *Eur Arch Otorhinolaryngol* 2004;261(1):6-24.

3   Jung JY, Chole RA. Bone resorption in chronic otitis media: the role of the osteoclast. *ORL J Otorhinolaryngol Relat Spec* 2002;64:95-107.

4   Kemppainen HO, Puhakka HJ, Laippala PJ, Sipila MM, Manninen MP, Karma PH. Epidemiology and aetiology of middle ear cholesteatoma. *Acta Otolaryngol* 1999;119:568-72.

5   Rosenfeld RM, Moura RL, Bluestone CD. Predictors of residual-recurrent cholesteatoma in children. *Arch Otolaryngol Head Neck Surg* 1992;118:384-91.

6   Sheahan P, Donnelly M, Kane R. Clinical features of newly presenting cases of chronic otitis media. *J Laryngol Otol* 2001;115:962-6.

7   Wetmore RF, Konkle DF, Potsic WP, Handler SD. Cholesteatoma in the pediatric patient. *Int J Pediatr Otorhinolaryngol* 1987;14:101-12.

8   Smith JA, Danner CJ. Complications of chronic otitis media and cholesteatoma. *Otolaryngol Clin North Am* 2006;39:1237-55.

9   Nunez DA, Browning GG. Risks of developing an otogenic intracranial abscess. *J Laryngol Otol* 1990;104:468-72.

10   Bain J, Williamson I. Treating the discharging ear in general practice. *BMJ* 1988;296:1617.

11   Syed I, Bhutta M. Facial nerve palsy: assessment and management. *Br J Hosp Med (Lond)* 2008;69(3):M34-7.

12   Milroy CM, Slack RW, Maw AR, Bradfield JW. Aural polyps as predictors of underlying cholesteatoma. *J Clin Pathol* 1989;42:460-5.

13   Lemmerling MM, de Foer B, VandeVyver V, Vercruysse JP, Verstraete KL. Imaging of the opacified middle ear. *Eur J Radiol* 2008;66:363-71.

14   Vercruysse JP, de Foer B, Somers T, Casselman J, Offeciers E. Magnetic resonance imaging of cholesteatoma: an update. *B-ENT* 2009;5:233-40.

15   O'Reilly BJ, Chevretton EB, Wylie I, Thakkar C, Butler P, Sathanathan N, et al. The value of CT scanning in chronic suppurative otitis media.
      J Laryngol Otol 1991;105:990-4.

16   Omran A, De Denato G, Piccirillo E, Leone O, Sanna M. Petrous bone cholesteatoma: management and outcomes. *Laryngoscope* 2006;116:619-26.

17   Ikeda M, Nakazato H, Onoda K, Hirai R, Kida A. Facial nerve paralysis caused by middle ear cholesteatoma and effects of surgical intervention. *Acta Otolaryngol* 2006;126:95-100.

18   Siddiq MA, Hanu-Cernat LM, Irving RM. Facial palsy secondary to cholesteatoma: analysis of outcome following surgery. *J Laryngol Otol* 2007;121:114-7.

More titles in
The BMJ Series

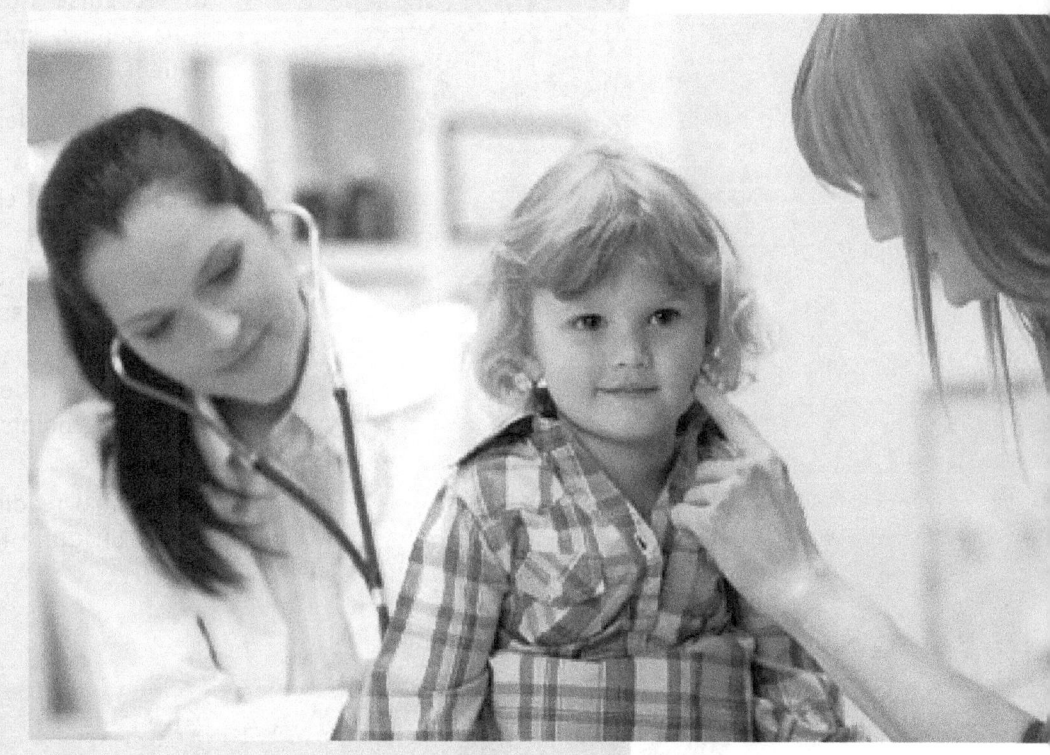

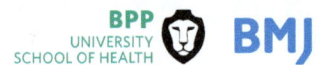
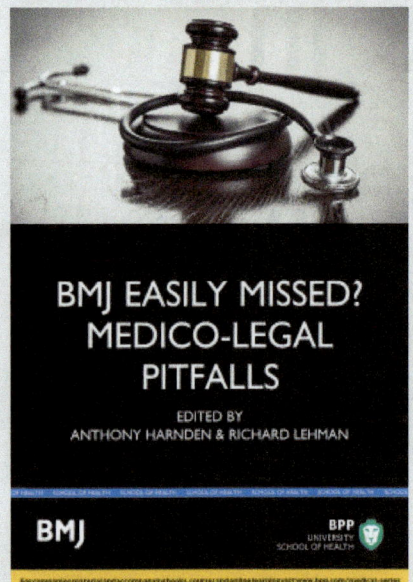
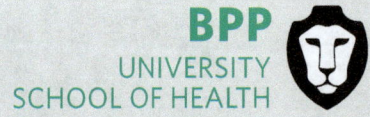

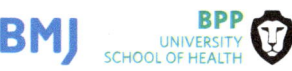
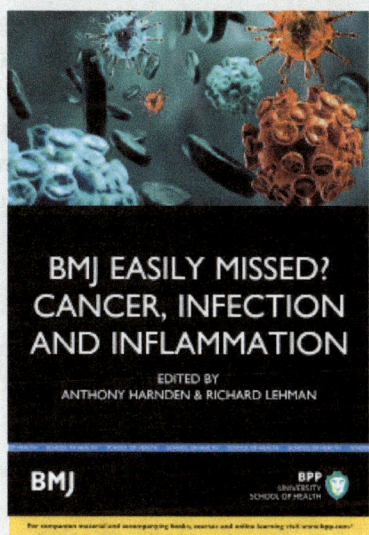
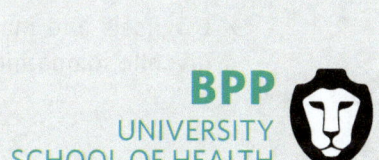

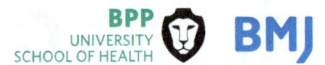
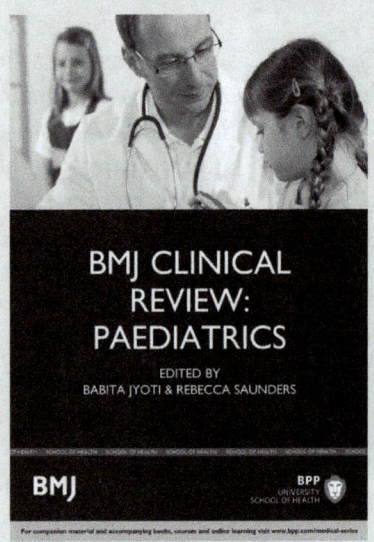
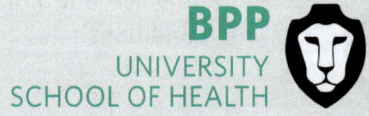

More titles from BPP School of Health

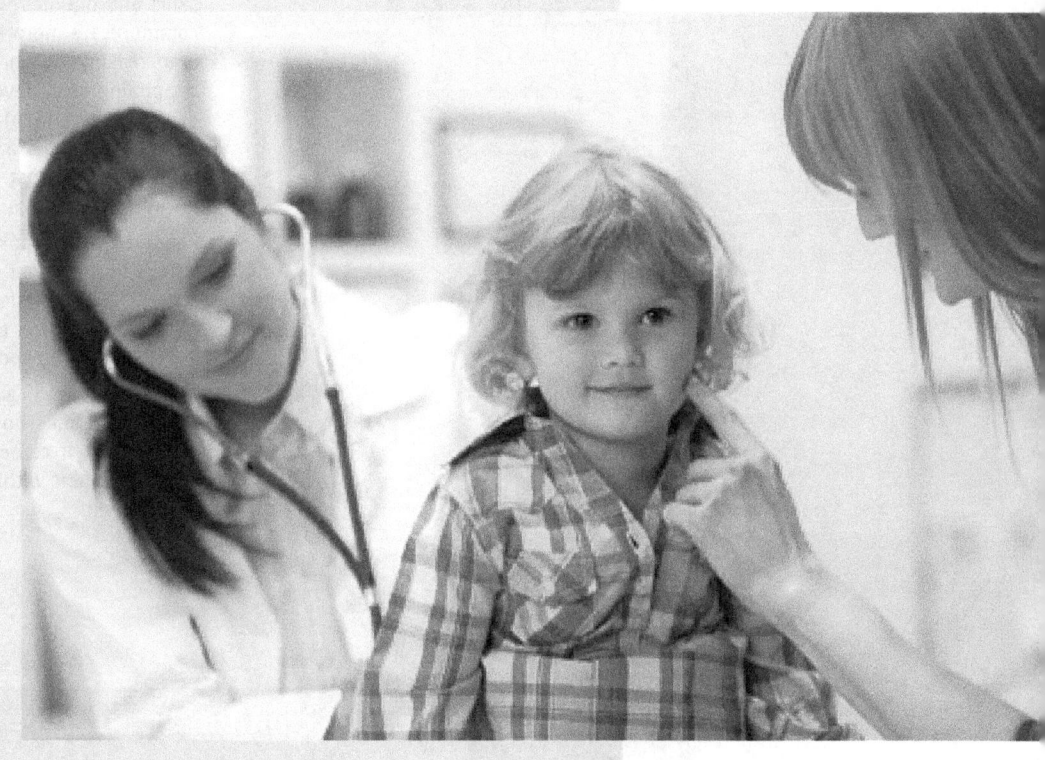

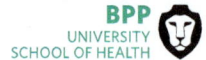
More titles in The Progressing your Medical Career Series

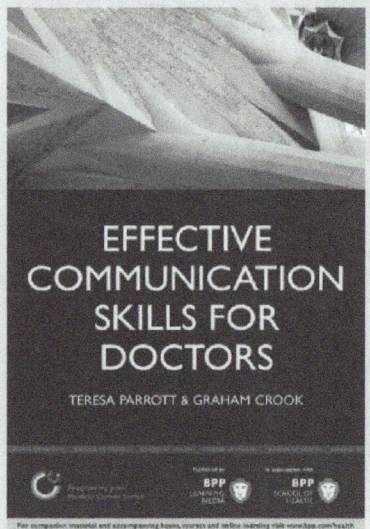

EFFECTIVE
COMMUNICATION
SKILLS FOR
DOCTORS

TERESA PARROTT & GRAHAM CROOK

£19.99
September 2011
Paperback
978-1-445379-56-2

Would you like to know how to improve your communication skills? Are you looking for a clearly written book which explores all aspects of effective medical communication?

There is an urgent need to improve doctors' communication skills. Research has shown that poor communication can contribute to patient dissatisfaction, lack of compliance and increased medico-legal problems. Improved communication skills will impact positively on all of these areas.

The last fifteen years have seen unprecedented changes in medicine and the role of doctors. Effective communication skills are vital to these new roles. But communication is not just related to personality. Skills can be learned which can make your communication more effective, and help you to improve your relationships with patients, their families and fellow doctors.

This book shows how to learn those skills and outlines why we all need to communicate more effectively. Healthcare is increasingly a partnership. Change is happening at all levels, from government directives to patient expectations. Communication is a bridge between the wisdom of the past and the vision of the future.

Readers of this book can also gain free access to an online module which upon successful completion can download a certificate for their portfolio of learning/Revalidation/CPD records.

This easy-to-read guide will help medical students and doctors at all stages of their careers improve their communication within a hospital environment.

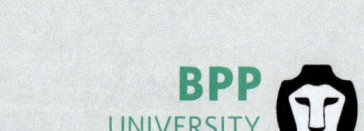

BPP
UNIVERSITY
SCHOOL OF HEALTH

www.bpp.com/medical-series

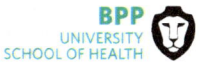

More titles in The Progressing your Medical Career Series

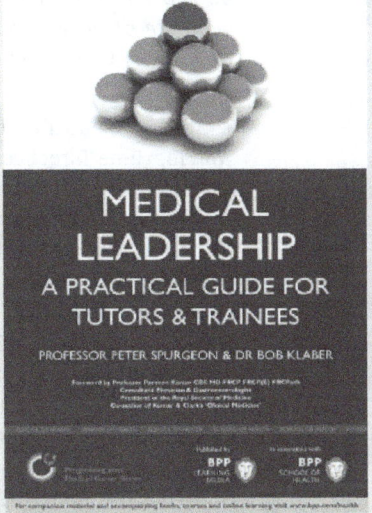

£19.99

November 2011

Paperback

978-1-445379-57-9

Are you a doctor or medical student who wishes to acquire and develop your leadership and management skills? Do you recognise the role and influence of strong leadership and management in modern medicine?

Clinical leadership is something in which all doctors should have an important role in terms of driving forward high quality care for their patients. In this up-to-date guide Peter Spurgeon and Robert Klaber take you through the latest leadership and management thinking, and how this links in with the Medical Leadership Competency Framework. As well as influencing undergraduate curricula and some of the concepts underpinning revalidation, this framework forms the basis of the leadership component of the curricula for all medical specialties, so a practical knowledge of it is essential for all doctors in training.

Using case studies and practical exercises to provide a strong work-based emphasis, this practical guide will enable you to build on your existing experiences to develop your leadership and management skills, and to develop strategies and approaches to improving care for your patients.

This book addresses:

- Why strong leadership and management are crucial to delivering high quality care
- The theory and evidence behind the Medical Leadership Competency Framework
- The practical aspects of leadership learning in a wide range of clinical environments (eg handover, EM, ward etc)
- How Consultants and trainers can best facilitate leadership learning for their trainees and students within the clinical work-place

Whether you are a medical student just starting out on your career, or an established doctor wishing to develop yourself as a clinical leader, this practical, easy-to-use guide will give you the techniques and knowledge you require to excel.

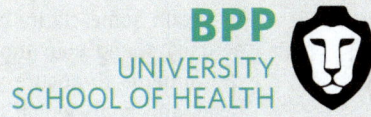

www.bpp.com/medical-series

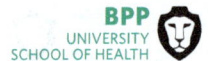
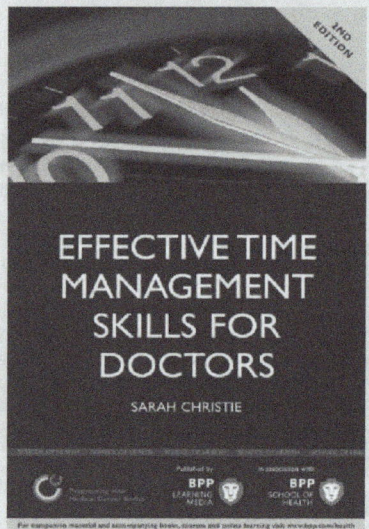
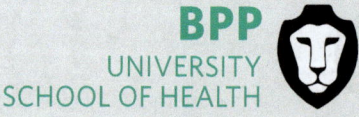

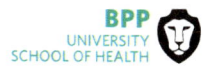

More titles in The Essential Clinical Handbook Series

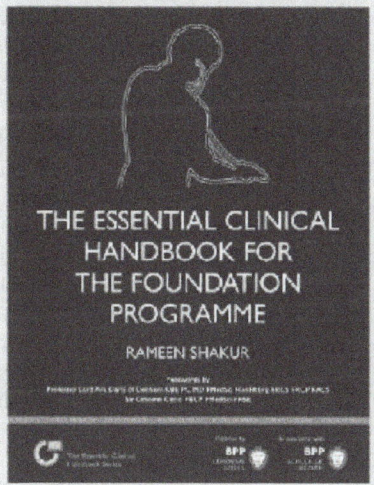

THE ESSENTIAL CLINICAL HANDBOOK FOR THE FOUNDATION PROGRAMME

RAMEEN SHAKUR

£24.99

October 2011

Paperback

978-1-445381-63-3

Unsure of what clinical competencies you must gain to successfully complete the Foundation Programme? Unclear on how to ensure your ePortfolio is complete to enable your progression to ST training?

This up-to-date clinical handbook is aimed at current foundation doctors and clinical medical students and provides a comprehensive companion to help you in the day-to-day management of patients on the ward. Together with this it is the first handbook to also outline clearly how to gain the core clinical competencies required for successful completion of the Foundation Programme. Written by doctors for doctors this comprehensive handbook explains how to successfully manage all of the common cases you will face during the Foundation Programme and:

- Introduces the Foundation Programme and what is expected of a new doctor especially with the introduction of Modernising Medical Careers

- Illustrates clearly the best way to manage, step-by-step, over 150 commonly encountered clinical diseases, including NICE guidelines to ensure a gold standard of clinical care is achieved.

- Describes how to successfully gain the core clinical competencies within Medicine and Surgery including an extensive list of differentials and conditions explained

- Explores the various radiology images you will encounter and how to interpret them

- Tells you how to succeed in the assessment methods used including DOP's, Mini-CEX's and CBD's

- Has step by step diagrammatic guide to doing common clinical procedures competently and safely.

- Outlines how to ensure your ePortfolio is maintained properly to ensure successful completion of the Foundation Programme.

- Provides tips and advice on how to start preparing now to ensure you are fully prepared and have the competitive edge for your CMT/ST application.

The introduction of the e-Portfolio as part of the Foundation Programme has paved the way for foundation doctors to take charge of their own learning and portfolio. Through following the expert guidance laid down in this handbook you will give yourself the best possible chance of progressing successfully through to CMT/ST training.

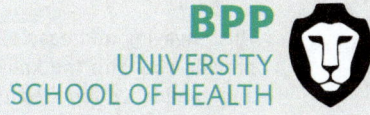

BPP
UNIVERSITY
SCHOOL OF HEALTH

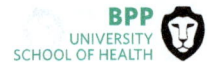

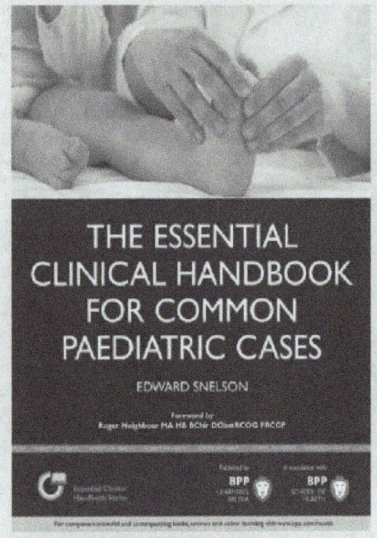
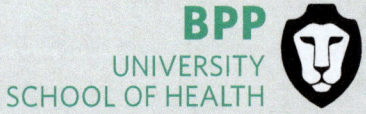

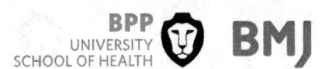

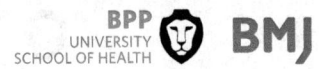